Personality
In Peptic Ulcer

Personality
In Peptic Ulcer

By

Albert J. Sullivan, M.D.

Head of Section on Gastroenterology, Ochsner Clinic, and Lecturer
in Medicine, Tulane University of Louisiana School of Medicine.
Formerly, Associate Clinical Professor of Medicine, Yale University
School of Medicine; Adjunct Clinical Professor of Medicine, George-
town University School of Medicine and George Washington University
School of Medicine

and

Thomas E. McKell, M.D.

Member of Section on Gastroenterology, Ochsner Clinic, and Instructor
in Medicine, Tulane University of Louisiana School of Medicine

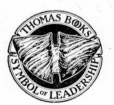

CHARLES C THOMAS · PUBLISHER

Springfield · Illinois · U.S.A.

CHARLES C THOMAS · PUBLISHER

BANNERSTONE HOUSE
301-327 EAST LAWRENCE AVENUE, SPRINGFIELD, ILLINOIS, U.S.A.

Published simultaneously in The British Commonwealth of Nations by
BLACKWELL SCIENTIFIC PUBLICATIONS, LTD., OXFORD

Published simultaneously in Canada by
THE RYERSON PRESS, TORONTO

FIRST EDITION

Printed in the United States of America

Introduction

Because the observations of internists, gastroenterologists, physiologists, surgeons and psychiatrists concerning the mechanism responsible for the production of peptic ulcer have multiplied in recent years, it seems desirable to correlate these into a unified picture. This monograph represents such an attempt. A theory of the production of peptic ulcer on the basis of multiple etiologic factors will be offered. Since our present day knowledge is not complete, this theory cannot be the final answer to such a complex problem. As our knowledge increases through improved methods of observation, a more inclusive explanation may be forthcoming.

Among our reasons for attempting to explain the mechanism of peptic ulcer is the fact that it is one of the commonest of all psychosomatic diseases, affecting at least 10 per cent of the population; an understanding of this disease is therefore essential to every practicing physician. Moreover, there is need for more discussion, evaluation and correlation of current observations concerning peptic ulcer and wider dissemination of this information among practicing physicians. It is further hoped that this study might be of value in the elucidation of other psychosomatic disorders which occur less frequently and in which investigations have been less numerous.

This study is based on clinical observations of both the psychic and somatic aspects of over 1000 cases of peptic ulcer. Unfortunately, a statistical review of these cases has not been possible because the patients were seen in a number of different cities and consequently their records are not available for detailed analysis. However, the last 200 cases have been analyzed and the results are consistent with the general impression obtained from our clinical experience with all patients with peptic ulcer.

Preface

A BOOK of this size can, of course, contain scarcely more than an outline of the personality in peptic ulcer. We have purposely refrained from a technical and encyclopedic discussion of the treatment of peptic ulcer because we are of the opinion that at this early stage in the development of psychosomatic medicine clarity and simplicity are of more value than profundity. Since much of contemporary psychologic medicine has yet to emerge from a fog of semantics, we have enlisted the help of a few visual aids.

We wish to express our sincere appreciation to numerous friends and colleagues whose helpful suggestions have been incorporated into these pages. Our special gratitude goes to Miss Selma de Bakey, Medical Editor of the *Alton Ochsner Medical Foundation,* whose numerous revisions of the text produced order out of chaos; to Dr. Frederick C. Rehfeldt, whose suggestions and facile crayon made our illustrations possible; to Mr. Harry De Vore of the *Cutawl Advertising Studio* in New Orleans, whose enthusiasm and genius gave three dimensions to our "characters"; and, finally, to our publisher, *Charles C Thomas · Publisher,* whose kind cooperation and scholarly interest has made possible the publication of this material despite present day printing difficulties.

Albert J. Sullivan, M.D.
Thomas E. McKell, M.D.

Contents

Personality
In Peptic Ulcer

1

Emotional Factors in Peptic Ulcer

ALTHOUGH all historical references to the psychosomatic aspects of peptic ulcer will not be reviewed, no discussion can be adequate which neglects two significant contributions. The first was made by that astute physician, William Brinton (9). In 1857, after completing a study of 1100 previously published necropsies on patients with gastric ulcer, 100 personally observed necropsies and 150 living patients on whom he had made the diagnosis of gastric ulcer, he wrote the first book *On the Pathology, Symptoms and Treatment of Ulcer of the Stomach*. Most of his observations and recommendations have stood the test of the last ninety years, none more so than his statement, "Mental anxiety so frequently coincides with ulcer that we are fully entitled to regard it as a more or less immediate cause."

Approximately sixty years later Kaufmann (32) read a paper before the American Gastroenterological Association entitled, *The Psychic Element as an Important Factor in the Development and Treatment of Peptic Ulcer*. This significant contribution has never received the attention it deserved. From clinical observations Kaufmann recognized that psychic influences, such as great emotional display, nervous shock and unduly prolonged or intense mental strain, play a prominent role in the development of peptic ulcer. He realized

3

that patients with peptic ulcer are usually high strung, excitable persons, prone to indulge in overactivity, and lead active lives. He observed that an emotional upset regularly preceded the periods of active gastric symptoms in his patients. Although he made no attempt to explain the physiologic mechanism whereby psychic influences are active in the formation of peptic ulcers, he emphasized the necessity for taking into consideration these influences in outlining a plan of treatment. Whether medical or surgical treatment was indicated, he believed that recurrences could largely be prevented by eliminating these harmful psychic influences, particularly emotional excesses and faulty habits of mental activity, though this might require thorough revision of the mode of living even to a change of occupation. He cited a detailed case of a young lawyer who characteristically had repeated attacks of peptic ulcer with hemorrhage following the strain of conducting prolonged cases in court and remissions between cases when the stress and strain were removed and a medical regimen was followed. Kaufmann clearly understood that there was no single etiologic factor responsible for all peptic ulcers. It was his opinion that dietary indiscretion and excessive use of alcohol and tobacco as well as emotional influences needed to be taken into account and he emphasized the importance of considering all possible etiologic factors if a more lasting therapeutic response is to be obtained.

These opinions along with others had little or no effect on the general attitude of the medical profession toward the etiology and treatment of peptic ulcer. Hurst and Stewart (27) in their classic 544-page monograph, *Gastric and Duodenal Ulcer,* published in 1929, devoted only three sentences to the emotional factor in peptic ulcer. In the section on the pathogenesis of ulcer they wrote, "The first appearance of symptoms of duodenal ulcer often follows a period of combined physical and mental overwork especially if it has been accompanied by worry. Still more frequently relapses and recurrences appeared to be precipitated in this way." In the chapter on symptoms they stated, "Overwork and worry often bring on attacks and in the early stages immediate relief may follow a week-end in the country or other congenial holiday away from work."

It is almost incredible that as late as the fourth decade of this century so little understanding of the psychogenic factors existed among clinicians. However, in the early years of this decade widespread interest in this field developed. Perhaps the three most significant contributions were made by Cushing (14), who again directed attention to the neurogenic mechanisms through which gastric erosions and perforations are occasionally produced by a cerebral lesion; by Alexander (2), who clearly stated his views of the psychogenic mechanisms involved; and by Draper and Touraine (18), whose studies on both the constitutional and emotional factors were of fundamental significance.

Others (11) investigating another psychosomatic affection, ulcerative colitis, were impressed by the contrast in personality of patients with this disease and those with peptic ulcer. Robinson (41) gave an excellent description of the usual ulcer personality in 1937 and in the same year Davies and Wilson (15) made an important contribution. By 1940 it was unusual to see an article on peptic ulcer which did not make some reference to psychic factors. However, still too wide a breach existed between the specialized knowledge available on the emotional factors in peptic ulcer and its understanding and use by the practicing physician.

The presentation of Alexander's hypothesis in 1934 was a great stimulus to those interested in the field of psychosomatic gastrointestinal problems. Alexander believed that the infant's wish to be taken care of and loved is gratified by the act of receiving milk at the mother's breast. Thus, the emotional qualities of receptivity become closely associated with the physiologic functions of nutrition; being fed becomes the primordial symbol of being loved. However, if this intense wish to be loved and to depend upon others is rejected by the adult ego and cannot find some other form of gratification, then only the regressive pathway remains, that is, the wish to be loved becomes converted into the wish to be fed. This repressed longing for love leads to stimulation of the stomach, for this wish to be fed is, of course, the primitive desire of the alimentary tract. This results in chronic stimulation of gastric function and leads to dysfunction, since gastric stimulation is independent of the normal conditioned stimulus—the need for food. The stomach, therefore, constantly acts as if it were receiving or about to receive food. The greater the rejection of every dependent desire in life, the greater becomes this unconscious wish for love and help. The patient wants food not because of organic hunger, but as a symbol of love and affection. Under this chronic stimulation the stomach behaves constantly as it ordinarily does during digestion. Chronic hypermotility and hypersecretion may thus be initiated. Chronic hypersecretion, chronic hunger pain and other symptoms are, therefore, the first indication that nervous control of gastric function has been disturbed. Alexander believed that psychotherapy is not only of considerable preventive value but it is also of great assistance when combined with medical therapy in managing the actual ulcer itself. He emphasized the significance of the psychoanalytic approach in such cases in view of the fact that peptic ulcers often develop in persons with deep-seated neurotic conflicts.

Alexander recognized that there is no single personality type characteristic of all patients with peptic ulcers. He believed that the characteristic feature is not so much the personality type as the fundamental conflict between receptive and active giving tendencies and attempts to abolish this conflict by overcompensation. The fact that all patients with ulcer do not fall into a single personality type is not unique in psychosomatic medicine. Dunbar (19) observed that 20 per cent of patients sustaining fractures do not fall into the "accident type" and that 15 to 20 per cent of patients with coronary occlusion are not the "coronary type" because they have hypertension and more closely resemble the "hypertensive type." Although our experience has shown that Alexander's theories apply to only a small number of patients with peptic ulcer, we find them indispensable in the daily practice of gastroenterology (particularly in anorexia nervosa, nervous vomiting, obesity and some types of diarrhea).

The primary objection to Alexander's theory of peptic ulcer is that it is based on a relatively small group of special cases, that is, patients with deep-seated neurosis. His hypothesis was formulated from a study of only nine cases (six cases of duodenal ulcer, only three of which were active at the time of psychoanalysis, and three of gastric neurosis). Most of the cases reported in the psychoanalytic literature obviously belong to this more neurotic group and these patients often have many other psychosomatic manifestations. We have been unable to find in the literature a single report of a patient with peptic ulcer who has undergone psychoanalysis and could be considered to have what we term a typical ulcer personality. In fact, it is difficult to conceive of a patient with the typical ulcer personality undergoing prolonged psychoanalysis for an ulcer since these patients are intolerant not only of medication and diet but also of prolonged psychiatric treatment.

Alexander's theory has been found to be applicable to only 11 per cent of our last 200 cases; it does not apply to the majority of patients with peptic ulcer, that is, those with the typical ulcer personality (72 per cent of our cases). If it did, these patients might be expected to be obese as the result of a voracious appetite. Actually, the reverse is true; the patient with the ulcer personality is not a glutton, is rarely obese, usually has less than the average appetite and tends to consider the whole business of eating of minor importance. Do these patients repress the desire to be loved, convert it into the wish to be fed and then reject that desire also?

As further evidence that a high percentage of patients with ulcer is not motivated by a deep-seated neurosis is the recent report on 162 hospitalized patients with ulcer studied by an internist and a psychiatrist (22). A psychiatric diagnosis was made on only 15 per cent of these patients, whereas statistically such a diagnosis is to be expected in 10 per cent of the population at large. Of the total of 25 psychiatric diagnoses, 13 or over half were anxiety neuroses. Obvious neurotic manifestations were not commonly encountered in their series. It was their impression that their patients as a whole were not being subjected to undue psychologic worries and that such stress as the patient did undergo was not dealt with in an inefficient or neurotic way. It was concluded that psychiatric treatment was needed in only a small proportion of cases of peptic ulcer.

2

Physiologic Transition from Emotion to Ulceration

In his original publication (2) and subsequently (4), Alexander made some remarkably accurate predictions of the physiologic mechanism whereby a chronic "wish to be fed" could lead to "chronic excitation of the stomach." The brilliant investigations at Cornell by Wolf, Wolff and Mittelmann (34, 50–52) have replaced theory with fact largely by means of direct observations through a permanent fistula into the stomach of their subject, "Tom." These experiments rank with those of Beaumont and indeed supplement them through recordings of the vascular, secretory and motor reactions of the stomach together with simultaneous observations on the emotional reactions to adverse experiences over relatively long periods of time.

In the experiments of Wolf and Wolff acid in small amounts was continuously secreted in the subject under basal conditions. Emotions such as fear and sadness, which involved a feeling of withdrawal, were accompanied by pallor of the gastric mucosa and inhibition of acid secretion and contraction. Objectively, the patient at this time would complain of lack of appetite and even nausea. Emotional conflicts involving anxiety, hostility and resentment were accompanied by hypersecretion, hypermotility, hyperemia and engorgement of the gas-

tric mucosa resembling hypertrophic gastritis. This series of events was associated with gastrointestinal
complaints such as heartburn and abdominal pain. Pro-
longation of emotional situations involving intense
anxiety, hostility and resentment was found to be accompanied by severe and prolonged engorgement,
hypermotility and hypersecretion. In this state, mucosal
erosions and hemorrhages were readily induced by even
the most trifling trauma and frequently bleeding points
appeared spontaneously as the result of vigorous con-
tractions of the wall of the stomach. Continuous contact of acid gastric juice with such a small eroded
surface in the mucous membrane resulted in accelerated
secretion of acid and further engorgement of the whole
mucosa. Prolonged exposure of such a lesion to acid
gastric juice resulted in the formation of a chronic ulcer
of the mucosa protruding through the abdominal fistula. Wolf and Wolff concluded that the chain of
events beginning with anxiety and conflict and the associated overactivity of the stomach and ending in
hemorrhage or perforation is the one involved in the
natural history of peptic ulcer in the human being.

Szasz and associates (48), impressed by the role of
hostility in the pathogenesis of peptic ulcer, recently
reported some exceedingly interesting observations on a
rather neurotic young man with a duodenal ulcer. They
demonstrated that anger stimulated the production of a
large volume of hydrochloric acid in this patient, that
this excessive secretion of hydrochloric acid could be
obtained even after a period of complete inhibition of
gastric acidity by the parenteral injection of enterogastrone, and that this stimulating effect of anger on

the secretion of hydrochloric acid could be abolished by bilateral vagus section.

From the psychosomatic viewpoint, these investigations have advanced our knowledge of the etiology and pathogenesis of peptic ulcer in several important respects. First, by a carefully controlled series of experiments it has definitely been shown that certain emotional conflicts, chiefly anxiety, will produce physiologic responses in the stomach which are favorable to the production of ulcer and that under these circumstances the slightest trauma will produce erosions and hemorrhages. They have thus helped to prove Alexander's contention that chronic excitation of the stomach by emotional tension is the mechanism by which ulcer is produced. Secondly, they have shown that such physiologic hyperactivity of the stomach can be demonstrated in patients with peptic ulcer (34). Thirdly, they have shown that such emotional conflicts are usually demonstrable in patients with ulcer particularly at the time of recurrence of symptoms (34). Finally, they have demonstrated that these conflicts, chiefly anxiety,* hostility, resentment and insecurity, need not necessarily be due to the subject's intense dependent desires but may be on a much more nonspecific basis. Although Alexander's hypothesis adequately explains the tensions, anxieties and frustrations in patients with intense dependent or receptive tendencies, Wolf and Wolff (51) have clearly shown that their subject manifested the same type of gastric hyperactivity when he reacted according to his own personality to many of the ordinary life situations which produce anxiety, hostility, resentment and frus-

---

*In our experience anxiety has been the one emotional response consistently present in the ulcer of psychosomatic origin.

tration. Their subject with the permanent gastric fistula was not an intensely neurotic person, did not have the typical ulcer personality and had never had a spontaneous peptic ulcer.

3

Theory of Multiple Etiology

ALTHOUGH peptic ulcer is now rather widely accepted as a psychosomatic affection (25), there are still
two diametrically opposed ideas regarding this disease
expressed in the literature. There are those who deny the
importance of the emotions because they see patients
with peptic ulcer without any obvious emotional disturbances. Others are so enthusiastic about the psychologic aspects of this disease that they attribute everything to the emotional stresses and strains (or "the
intense dependent desires") and ignore the organic
factors. Although the latter group freely uses the term
"psychosomatic," in its enthusiasm for the new (the
psychic) it has discarded all the known facts concerning the old (the organic) which have been slowly and
carefully accumulated during the past century. The
formula to be presented may serve to reconcile even
these two extreme viewpoints; it makes allowance for
the fact that not only has it been proved that many
different factors are concerned in the production of
ulcer but in most instances the lesion is produced by
several factors varying in kind and degree from patient
to patient. This formula also allows for the characteristic recurrences of peptic ulcer.

One of us previously expressed the opinion that peptic ulcer is produced not by one etiologic factor but rather by a combination of many factors varying in their respective importance in each case. This was expressed in the form of an algebraic equation (6).

This formula has been gradually modified until it now reads

$$u = \frac{a + b + c + d + x^*}{r}$$

Where

u = the peptic ulcer (esophageal, gastric, duodenal or anastomotic),

a = constitutional (18) and genetic factors,

b = the predisposing personality or the intrinsic psychic factors,

c = the acute precipitating emotional situations or the extrinsic psychologic factors,

d = trauma which may be internal (food, condiments, or alcohol), external (a violent blow on the upper part of the abdomen), or intrinsic (gastrospasm),

x = all the physiologic and pathologic factors which are unique in producing an ulcer rather than cardiospasm, ulcerative colitis, asthma or some other psychosomatic affection. They may be *essential* to the production of ulcer, such as the presence of hydrochloric acid and pepsin or only *incidental,* such as local tissue allergy (Shwartzmann phenomenon) (13). They may be *local,* such as the exhaustion of mucous secretion or *systemic,*

$^*u$ = ulcer

a = constitution

b = personality

r = resistance

c = precipitating situation

d = trauma

x = unique factors

such as the shock from a burn which produces a fall in blood pressure and anoxia resulting in Curling's ulcer. They may be *well understood,* such as the ulcer produced by the pharmacologic action of histamine given for the treatment of headache (28) or *poorly understood,* such as the absence of those factors apparently supplied by the parenteral injection of enterogastrone. They may be *vascular* from thrombosis or an infected embolus, or *neurogenic,* such as the gastric lesions which follow injuries to the brain or spinal cord. Equally important are those neurogenic impulses which are severed by vagotomy.

Finally, *r* is a constant which represents the natural resistance of living gastroduodenal mucosa to peptic digestion. Alexander (3) recently suggested that a formula similar in part to this one might be used in most of the psychosomatic affections.

To facilitate discussion of the algebraic possibilities of this equation numerical values have been arbitrarily assigned to some parts of the equation, since the various factors in the formula cannot as yet be measured accurately enough to assign exact values to them. It may be assumed that *r* is a constant "figure 1" or unity and that it is the same for all individuals. This is certainly possible, for gastric mucosa possesses a certain innate ability to resist peptic digestion (38) which is greater than that of any other tissue in the body and, as far as we know, this resistance may be essentially the same in all human beings. Although this resistance may, of course, be overcome by a preponderance of one or more of the factors in the numerator, it is of such quality that even when these factors are present in normal quantities ulcers develop in relatively few people.

U must also be given a value of 1, that is, to break down gastric mucosa or to form an ulcer the equation must be balanced. *U,* which is 1, must also be balanced by 1 on the opposite side of the equation; in other words mucosal breakdown occurs when the factors tending to produce an ulcer reach an intensity of 1.

Factors *a, b, c, d* and *x* may be given any arbitrary fractional values provided their sum is less than 1 in a normal person without an ulcer. The equation can now be used in the understanding of peptic ulcer in most of its protean aspects.

The application of this equation may be illustrated by the hypothetical case of a 19-year-old boy whose father has been suffering from a peptic ulcer for years. The patient, however, has never had any significant gastric symptoms. He is of the ulcer habitus (factor *a*); he has the ulcer personality (factor *b*); his chief cells can secrete considerable hydrochloric acid (one of the *x* factors) and perhaps even tend to pour out more at night than those of the normal person. However, factor *c* is absent since there have been no acute emotional precipitating situations in his life and factor *d* (trauma to the gastric or duodenal mucosa) has been minimal. A peptic ulcer has not developed in this patient because the sum of the factors in the numerator of this equation is, let us say, 0.6 or 0.7.

At the age of 20 years when the boy's father is killed in an accident, the patient has to assume great economic responsibility which necessitates his leaving school, taking a difficult job and supplementing his income by selling life insurance in the evening. He also has to settle his father's estate, plan for the education of his younger brothers and comfort his mother. During the next few months symptoms begin to appear but they disappear when he modifies his diet. In a month or two they recur but still are not severe enough to consult a physician. At this point the sum of the factors in the numerator has reached 1.0 or 1.1. An ulcer develops but after the patient modifies his activities sufficiently, the total of these factors may drop to 0.9 and the ulcer heals.

A year later the patient is drafted for military service. While in training camp he has to live on food ill prepared by home standards. A few more symptoms appear but he does not report on sick call. Soon he is overseas exposed to K rations, alcohol, inclement weather and the constant threat of combat. The sum of factors a, b, c, d, and x by this time may be well over 1.0; it may reach 1.3, for example, and the symptoms are typical and severe. Merely modification of diet and neutralization of excessive hydrochloric acid with an antacid may still be enough to reduce the sum of the factors to 0.8 or 0.9 with consequent rapid healing. If, however, the total of the factors has reached 1.4, for example, other therapeutic agents must be employed. In addition to diet and alkali which modify only factors d and x, it might be necessary to use sedation and to supply rest in bed in a base hospital, which would modify factors b and c. It might even be necessary to alter these factors by discharge from the Army. If the sum of the factors is unusually high, 1.6 for instance, medical treatment may be unavailing and hemorrhage or perforation may occur. If the sum reaches 2.0 or some correspondingly high figure, surgical treatment, which modifies the x factors particularly may be necessary. Such procedures as pylorectomy or gastrojejunostomy, which do not affect the *x* factors to a great degree, may be followed by anastomotic ulcers and further surgical measures may be necessary.

This equation, based on multiple etiologic factors, not only explains the production but also the characteristic recurrences of peptic ulcers. Therapy such as diet, antacids or modifications in the life situation, by decreasing the numerator reduces the figure to less than 1 and healing occurs, whereas indiscretions in diet or the stresses and strains of life may increase it to greater than 1 and result in recurrence.

The evaluation of the life history of a patient in terms of this formula is a fascinating study. The numerator of the equation is the sum of many factors, several of which may be slight or entirely absent. Such low values in some factors must be balanced by corresponding increases in the remaining factors in order for an ulcer to develop. The constitutional factor was absent or negligible in about 40 per cent of our last 200 cases of peptic ulcer. A specific "ulcer personality" was present in only 72 per cent of these cases. The acute precipitating emotional situation was severe in only 10 to 15 per cent of cases. If factors *a, b,* and *c* are absent, the ulcer itself may be an unusual one, that is, it may be a gastric ulcer or an acute erosion; it may occur only on one occasion or the usual "food-ease-pain" rhythm may be absent.

Aaron (1) once related the life history of a patient with peptic ulcer who had undergone an almost incredible series of recurrences, hemorrhages, perforations and numerous surgical procedures finally ending in total gastrectomy only to have the patient succumb later to a perforating peptic ulcer of the esophagus! The relative importance of factors a, b, c, d, and x and the unusual degree which some of them must have reached in such a patient would have made an interesting study.

4

Clinical Classification of Cases

THE constitutional and genetic factors (*a* in our formula), trauma (*d*) and the *x* factors will not be analyzed in any detail. This discussion will be concerned primarily with factors *b* (the personality) and *c* (the precipitating situation). Of course, all etiologic factors are interdependent and cannot be completely compartmentalized. For example, given the ulcer personality and a precipitating situation in the form of a severe business reversal, the ensuing flare-up of symptoms cannot be attributed solely to the emotional factor, for in throwing himself into his work, in his hectic eighteen-to-twenty-hour workday, in his insomnia and dreams the patient provides continuous nocturnal secretion of acid (an *x* factor); he goes long hours between feedings, he bolts his food down instead of masticating properly (trauma); he may consume many cups of coffee or bottles of iced cold drinks. Roth and Ivy (43) recognized this when they stated, "a substrate of psychosomatic personality plus 10 to 15 cups of coffee may bring an ulcer." For a brilliant series of experiments on the multiple etiologic factors (largely *x* factors) necessary to produce ulcer in animals the reader is referred to the investigations of Wangensteen (49). Some of his experiments clearly showed that many separate pathogenic factors can be demonstrated.

Considerable clinical investigation remains to be done on the interrelation between factors; for example, are not many aspects of personality (*b*) and *x* factors such as high acid secretion related and may not both be inherited? In many cases they may be but in others such a relation may be absent. We have seen a person in the sixth decade of life who had the typical ulcer personality all his life, but never had an ulcer. His mother had died of pernicious anemia and he had no free hydrochloric acid even after the administration of histamine.

Since this study is not primarily concerned with the constitutional, traumatic or *x* factors, the 200 cases which have been analyzed were classified into the following four groups. Group A, the largest group (72 per cent of cases) consisted of patients with the "typical ulcer personality." Patients in Group B (11 per cent) were definitely psychoneurotic. In Group C (5 per cent) there was some striking external precipitating situation (factor *c*) and in Group D (10 per cent) there were no intrinsic (personality) or extrinsic (situational) psychic factors but there was some unusual degree of factors *a, d* or *x*. The remaining 2 per cent probably represented incomplete observations on our part. Either a satisfactory history was not obtained or the patients withheld or forgot relevant information so that they could not be correctly classified in one of the four groups.

5

The Ulcer Personality

THE ulcer personality (Group A) as it is seen in the clinic or consulting room will be discussed in the ensuing pages in non-psychiatric terms so that it may be easily recognized by others who, like ourselves, have had no formal psychiatric training. The way these patients react to many every day life situations will be particularly emphasized.

Drive

The ulcer patient is the tense, anxious, driving, active, mildly agitated individual frequently seen as the go-getter, the promoter, the organizer, the manager, the executive, the business man who cannot seem to let up, who will not admit defeat and who is continually striving to excel in his environment, who cannot relax or drift with the tide but must fight upstream against the current which would deposit him in the eddies or backwaters of life. It has long been known that there is a higher incidence of peptic ulcer in bus drivers, taxi drivers, railroad engineers and others who by their occupations express tremendous "drive." We once had a dispensary patient, who, when asked his occupation, said he "drove" an engine but actually he was a stationary engineer who ran a donkey engine. Often these patients take positions such as traveling salesmen be-

cause they "like to be on the go." Perhaps, as suggested
by Alexander, this drive comes from a repressed tendency; even so, the resultant hyperactivity itself creates
a restlessness, tension and anxiety which are in turn relieved only by more activity. "I must always be on the
go; I feel better when I am doing something" is often
expressed by patients.

This compulsive quality of activity in patients with
peptic ulcer was brought out in a comparative study of
the personality of 205 patients with ulcer and 100 patients with hernia of comparable age, sex, class and
source made by Davies and Wilson (15). This trait was
noted in 58 per cent of their patients with peptic ulcer
and only 14 per cent of those with hernia.

Brown (12) noted in a given combat situation in the
Pacific that the soldier who was frustrated and
"couldn't do anything about it" was the one who had
gastric symptoms. For example, of two anti-aircraft
gunners being bombed by the Japanese, the one whose
high-ranged gun could reach the altitude at which the
Japanese planes were flying and who was busily engaged
in firing his gun would be free of gastric symptoms. The
neighboring gunner whose rifle was of low range and
useless against these particular planes would often complain of severe gastric symptoms. The latter might fire
his gun even though he knew it was useless because "it
made me feel better to be doing something."

Versatility

This intense desire always to be doing something
leads most patients with ulcer to hold many jobs at once,
to take part in many extracurricular activities, to acquire civic, political or other organizational outlets for

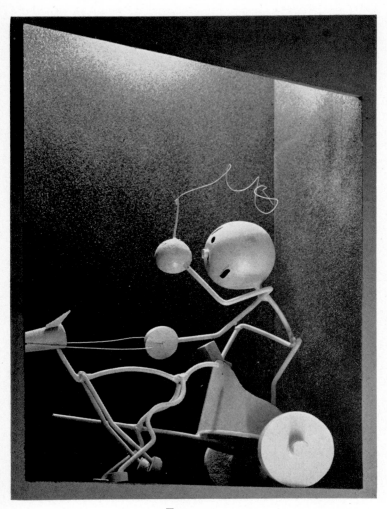

FIGURE 1

DRIVING

their drives and ambitions and to neglect to take vacations or long week-ends. There has been a common layman's expression in recent years that "there is at least one ulcer on every board of directors." Its corollary could well be that every ulcer patient is on several boards of directors. There will scarcely be a physician reading this who cannot recall a patient with peptic ulcer who is engaged in several professional activities combined with other responsibilities such as directorships and committee work and perhaps an active participation in some form of the arts. Such individuals are the rule, not the exception, and such versatility in activities is seen in the dispensary or charity ward as well as in the consulting room.

In 1934 with Dr. Warren Brown and John Dillon, a Yale Medical School student, one of us (A.J.S.) studied 15 consecutive patients with ulcer (by chance all were males) in the Gastrointestinal Clinic of the New Haven Dispensary. Of these, 13 had the typical ulcer personality. Three of these were officers in the labor unions of their trades, four were accomplished musicians who worked from two to four nights a week to earn extra money, nine were versatile enough to work at a half dozen different skills, one ran concessions at fairs during his vacations, one raised fancy poultry for sale and one caned chairs at night and on week-ends to earn extra money. There was one patient in that same dispensary not included in this group who worked as a laborer with a pick and shovel from 7:00 A.M. to 3:00 P.M., as an assistant in a florist shop from 3:30 P.M. until it closed at 8:00 P.M., then drove a cab at the railroad station until 12:00 or 1:00 A.M. and on week-ends made parachute jumps at county fairs.

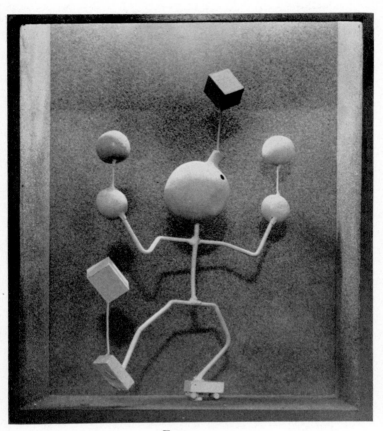

FIGURE 2

ACTIVE

It is interesting to observe patients with peptic ulcer on the wards of a charity hospital. In general they exhibit the same drive and restlessness. One of us once facetiously remarked, "Duodenal ulcers are often missed because the patients are never in their beds when the visiting physician makes rounds." On one occasion we (7) had four patients with ulcer on a charity ward, all with the typical ulcer personality. One was admitted in poor physical condition with almost complete pyloric obstruction; within forty-eight hours he had organized a baseball pool among the patients and was making about five dollars a day. The second could not lie in bed doing nothing so he worked six to eight hours a day in the pharmacy cleaning bottles. A third patient made arrangements with a friend to bring in boxes of candy bars which he sold the patients. A fourth made himself so useful to the nurses and internes that he was installed as an unofficial orderly and laboratory assistant.

Although a few questions as to the number of jobs and extracurricular activities in which the patient is engaged may be of great assistance in estimating the personality of the patient suspected of having an ulcer, it must be realized that this trait is frequently modified by circumstances and a wide knowledge of various occupations is necessary in order to elicit this information in some cases. Certain occupations, such as that of a traveling salesman, may require sixteen to eighteen hours daily and leave no time for outside activities. Farmers are often apparent but not true exceptions to the rule since they may work from before dawn until long after dusk; their drive may be expressed in an increasing effort to get more out of the farm by growing an extra crop, by raising poultry or other stock and by

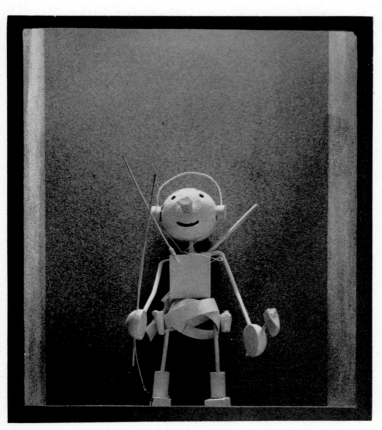

FIGURE 3

VERSATILE

ceaselessly trying to improve the home and farm build-
ings with repairs and additions. The farmer with a peptic ulcer, instead of relaxing a little in the few months
between growing seasons by doing a bit of fishing,
usually hires himself and his truck out, drives a school
bus or takes part in some other activity which will
"bring in some cash money."

With these drives and ambitions is it any wonder that
ulcer patients are usually successful? Those with the
typical ulcer personality always achieve some degree of
success at their own social, intellectual and economic
level. The ulcer patient may be only a janitor but he
will be the best janitor in his part of town and he will
have made himself invaluable to the tenants of his building by doing many things the average janitor would
never consider.

Emotional Responsiveness

Because these patients are usually pleasant persons
with whom rapport is good, they want their physician
to like them and they are likable. They will go out of
their way to be cooperative. They are continually trying to sell themselves. Draper (17) described their
emotional responsiveness as "swift and intent," and
considered them "by far the most dramatic personalities
on the medical and surgical wards."

Self Reliance

The ulcer personality is usually a striking example of
early emancipation from parental dependence. It is
not at all unusual to learn that as a child of 9, 10 or 12
years the patient with peptic ulcer assumed a position
as the head of the household. A recent patient of ours

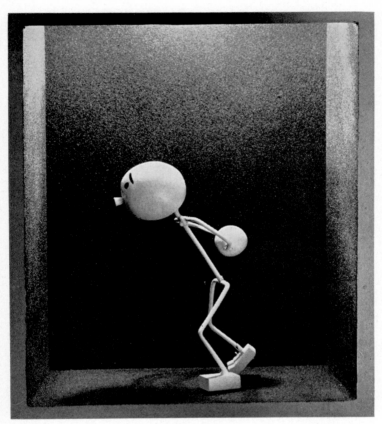

FIGURE 4

RESTLESS

at the age of 12 years was acting as head of the household, which consisted of his father, mother and six younger brothers and sisters. This patient would perform many of the chores on the farm in the early morning, would prepare breakfast, feed his father, the other children and then his mother, who was an invalid. He would then dress the younger children and before the sun had risen in the morning would walk nine miles to school. At the age of 13 he was recognized in the community as head of the household.

These patients frequently contribute significant amounts to the family treasury at an early age. They often leave the small communities in which they are born because of lack of opportunities, seeking new worlds to conquer. A recent patient of ours at the age of 15 years left his native land and went to a neighboring country where two much older brothers were unsuccessfully engaged in a business left by their deceased father. Our patient took charge of this business and within a year converted it to an overwhelming success.

Responsibility

Among the reasons for this early emancipation is the patient's own willingness to assume responsibility. Overly conscientious about responsibilities, these patients assume much more than their share. They make a constant effort to go more than half way with the other person. They want to be liked and thus indirectly to acquire a certain amount of confidence and security and this is one of the reasons why they will assume responsibility. In turn these added responsibilities result in a good deal of the tension, unrest and anxiety with which the ulcer patient eventually finds himself saddled. As

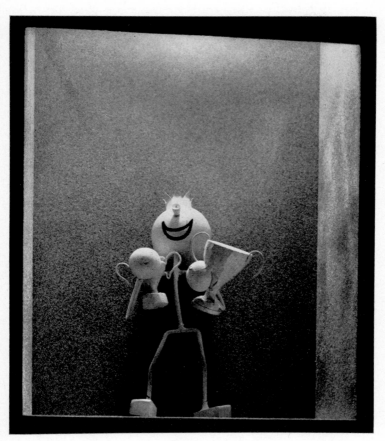

FIGURE 5

SUCCESSFUL

Davies and Wilson (15) so aptly expressed it, "Our investigations suggest that the ulcer individual is more liable to rebuffs and failures than his less ambitious, less active brother. Yet he is able to pass through life happily until some acute stress or anxiety is suddenly experienced, when he is liable to discharge his increased tension via special channels of his autonomic nervous system."

These patients carry their sense of responsibility into their family relationships, their social life and their business activities. They often assume the responsibility for the upbringing of the children of distant relatives. Rarely will they refuse the responsibilities which are thrust upon them in the way of committee work, chairmanships and directorships. They recognize that because of this they are often imposed upon. In their business activities they not only assume full responsibility for their own work but worry about the work of others; they are often rather overly precise and inclined to worry unduly over details and inevitable situations.

Sexual Adjustment

Ulcer patients usually make good heterosexual adjustment. They had the highest marriage (59 out of 62) and one of the lowest divorce (4 per cent) rates of any gastrointestinal disorder in a recent analysis of 500 cases (46). Davies and Wilson (15) observed that "Sexual problems are conspicuous by their relative absence and are only present when they relate to income and expenditure."

Determination

Another characteristic of the patient with the ulcer personality is his determined defiance of his environ-

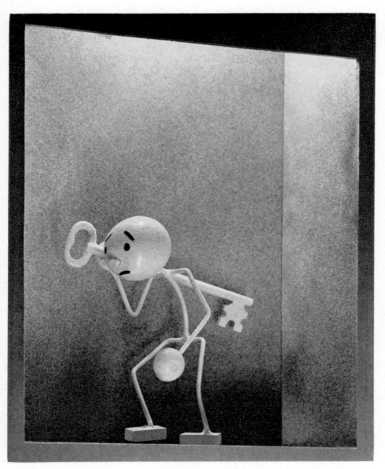

FIGURE 6

RESPONSIBLE

ment and illness. He refuses to surrender in the face of adversities. During business depressions, he will roll up his sleeves and redouble his activities. His reaction to his gastric discomfort is similar. He refuses to give up when his stomach starts to bother him; he does not make even minor concessions to diet.

One need only contrast the ulcer patient who refuses to give up even though he has been having tarry stools for three or four days and knows their significance with the reaction of a neurasthenic or hypochondriacal woman who takes to her bed because she sees a little mucus in her stool. We have even seen a patient with a perforated peptic ulcer continue working for another three hours until the day's work was completed before reporting to his doctor on his way home from work.

The average neurotic patient who enjoys his illness is the antithesis of the patient with the typical ulcer personality. This has been pointed out by Jones (30), who found little spread between perception of pain and reaction to pain in the neurotic patient, whereas in ulcer patients although the threshold of pain was normal the reaction to pain was at a much higher normal level.

Experiences of Halstead (26) among patients with gastric disorders in the Mediterranean theater also emphasize this point. There were about 500 cases of gastric neurosis or psychogenic dyspepsia as it was termed, and only 250 cases of peptic ulcer among 14,000 admissions to the hospital during a period of one year.

Halstead observed such a constant difference between the personality of patients with peptic ulcer and those with nonulcerative dyspepsia that an accurate diagnosis could be made from the history alone in about

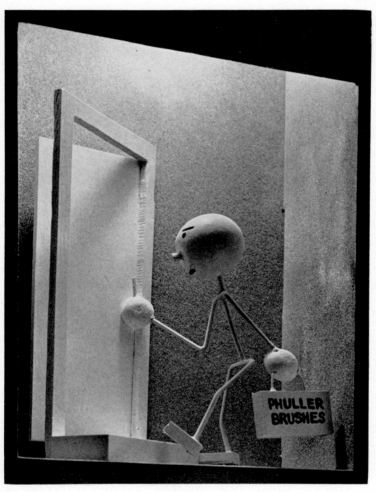

FIGURE 7

DETERMINED

90 per cent of cases. Psychiatric studies were conducted by Halstead on the neuropsychiatric service on 100 patients with ulcer and 100 with chronic nonulcerative dyspepsia. In the group without ulcers 80 per cent were psychoneurotic whereas in the group with ulcers only 6 per cent had disabilities resulting from a psychoneurosis.* On the other hand, Halstead observed that the incidence of neurotic traits, although considerable among the patients with ulcer, was not enough to disable them. The personality makeup of the patient with ulcer was described as that of a restless, ambitious individual intensely anxious to succeed. He was self-sufficient, self-reliant and usually an excellent soldier. Although a long history of continued indigestion could often be obtained, the man would rarely report this if he were in combat or in a difficult situation until he had finished his mission, whereas the patient with nonulcerative dyspepsia usually made use of his symptoms to avoid an unpleasant situation. The latter was often a habitue of sick call and typically a submissive, passive individual. Friedman (26a) has recently confirmed Halstead's observations.

Age

Age is of some significance in understanding peptic ulcer in terms of the personality. First, of course, it must be clearly understood that the ulcer personality manifests itself before the appearance of the disease and is not a result of the disease; it is not the cause of the ulcer but merely predisposes to the onset and re-

---

*These are cases which we would probably classify in Group B. Since this group of soldiers was screened several times before going overseas, this figure of 6 per cent corresponds fairly well with the 11 per cent which we classified in Group B.

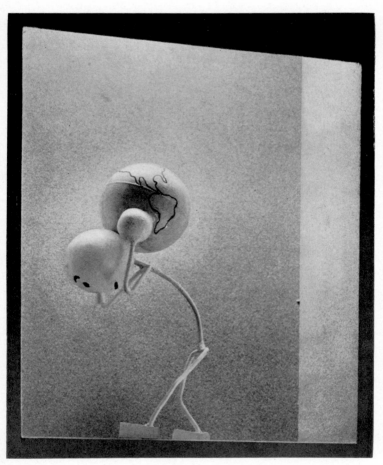

FIGURE 8

CONSCIENTIOUS

currences of the ulcer. There are different degrees of the ulcer personality. It may be obvious and require only a few simple questions to bring it out or in some instances it may be scarcely recognizable; that is, the patient may have only a few of the typical characteristics. It is probable that more persons have the ulcer personality than will be found to have peptic ulcers since the personality is not the sole cause of the ulcer.

In general, when the premorbid ulcer personality approaches the typical and is well defined, the disease tends to develop in the third decade of life because this is usually the period during which the patient is subjected to the greatest stresses and strains in his efforts to establish himself from the financial and domestic point of view and during which his drive is at its peak. This does not mean that he will necessarily consult a physician at this time; on the contrary, he may refuse to yield to his gastric symptoms for another five years or more.

It has been our experience that if the ulcer develops in the early part of the second decade of life, constitutional or genetic factors (*a*) are apt to be prominent (Case 18).* Alvarez (5) mentions "a husband and wife, both extremely nervous and their two sons, aged ten and twelve years," all of whom were found to have duodenal ulcers. Conversely, if an ulcer develops in a patient for the first time after the age of 50 years, the premorbid personality is usually not that of the ulcer type or at least not strongly so and other etiologic factors, such as acute precipitating emotional situations or vascular factors (49), may be of greater than usual importance.

*See Report of Cases, page 91.

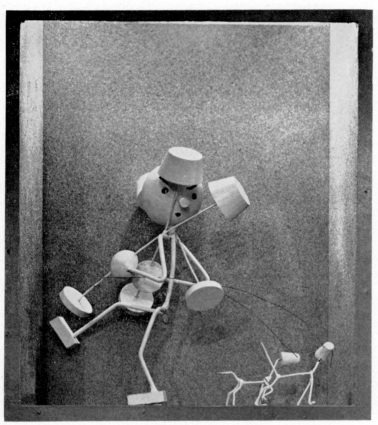

FIGURE 9

OVEREXTENDED

The work of Hall, Ettinger and Banting (24), who observed in giving infusions of acetylcholine to dogs, that retching, vomiting, hematemesis and melena developed only in the young dogs, gives experimental data suggesting that youth is more susceptible to gastric erosion.

It should also be remembered that the ulcer personality is often tempered by experience. By the time the patient reaches the age of 55 or 60 years he has usually begun to modify his drive. He may have reached a position which nearly satisfies his craving for success; he may have decided that he cannot change the world or his small part of it single-handedly or perhaps he has learned to appreciate other things than success, power and money. The mellowing effect of age seems definitely to reduce the frequency and severity of symptoms provided the ulcerative lesion has not produced permanent irreversible structural changes. It is interesting that this same beneficial effect of age is noted in many other psychosomatic affections (47). An estimate of the proportion of the total liability to peptic ulcer which has been survived by a given age has been tabulated (Table I, page 64) by Gainsborough and Slater (22).

Sex

The typical ulcer personality is seen in women with ulcers, but not as frequently as in men. The ulcer usually develops in the third decade in women, and almost invariably the patient is engaged in a business or profession at the onset of symptoms. If these women become housewives, the ulcer usually becomes quiescent, often permanently. Although the housewife has many daily tasks to perform, she is not exposed to the competition of the commercial world, or perhaps her desire for success is not personal but includes all members of the family. The professional woman who gives up her career is usually giving up independence for dependence in return, of course, for affection. Her freedom from further ulcer recurrences gives support to Alexander's theory. Occasionally, the married woman with an ulcer may have such a typical ulcer personality and be engaged in such outside activities as to make her the exact counterpart of the busy male executive (Case 2). In females with the ulcer personality the acute precipitating situation is usually concerned with reverses in financial matters or related to work and is not severe or dramatic. One not infrequently sees a woman who had ulcer symptoms while working before her marriage and whose symptoms remained quiescent during twenty years of marriage only to recur at the death of her husband when financial circumstances compelled the patient to support her family (Case 4). The rarity of active ulcers among married women has been commented upon by Sandweiss and associates (44), who found only one active ulcer among 70,000 consecutive pregnant women.

Race

It is commonly believed that the Negro is less susceptible to peptic ulcer than the white race; in fact, Robinson (41) in 1935 wrote, "The negro and lesser pigmented races are immune to the disease. The white race alone is susceptible." Rivers (40) is partially responsible for this erroneous impression despite the fact that his early description of the ulcer personality was excellent. He noted that among 200 specialists in medicine almost 20 per cent had peptic ulcers and another 20 per cent admitted taking alkalis at intervals especially during periods in which they were under unusual stress or strain. This high incidence of ulcer and gastric symptomatology was in striking contrast to the incidence among 200 Negroes living in a county seat in central Texas. Negroes of all types were deliberately chosen and most were the slow moving, easy going type untouched by aspiration for culture. Characteristically, the diet of these Negroes was not balanced and their habits almost invariably included the abuse of tobacco and alcohol. In general, they lived under pathetic hygienic conditions, they dissipated recklessly, their hours of sleep were entirely without regularity, and they ate whatever they could get. Many were without work and scarcely knew the source of the next day's food but even those with large families were surprisingly unconcerned about their difficulties. Yet the syndrome of peptic ulcer was rarely encountered among these Negroes. No instance of ulcer complicated by perforation, obstruction or hemorrhage was encountered and in only one case was there sufficient evidence in the history to make a diagnosis of peptic ulcer. Only 3 per cent of the Negroes had indigestion.

Whereas Rivers has shown that faulty diet, dissipation and the excessive use of tobacco and alcohol did not produce ulcer in the group of southern agricultural Negroes he studied, this could also be shown to be true in many selected groups, whether Negro or white. Moreover, Steigmann (45) showed conclusively that among Negroes in industrial areas in the North peptic ulcer is as common as among the white race and furthermore these Negroes are of the same general personality type.

One of the most striking examples of the ulcer personality that one of us has ever seen was in a Negro born in a southern Texas city who was left an orphan at an early age. At the age of nine years he ran away from his foster parents, crossed the border into Mexico and became a water boy for a construction company. He later became a professional baseball player on one of the best Negro professional baseball teams. Despite loss of a leg in a railroad accident, he took up professional swimming and diving. At the time we saw him he was considered the best pants presser in Washington, D.C. He would often work overtime to make more money. He was still drawing a small income from diving exhibitions, he served on many committees and was active in religious groups. He owned his own home and was constantly improving it.

Like the Negro, the Chinese (the phlegmatic race) have been considered immune to peptic ulcer. However, it has been shown that among the Chinese living with the Malays and controlling most of the little businesses in Java and Sumatra, the incidence of peptic ulcer is ten times as great as among the Malays themselves (8,36).

Geography

Peptic ulcer does not appear to be a matter of geography although it could probably be shown statistically that there are fewer cases of ulcer in small communities than in large ones or more in the North than in the South. It is our opinion that persons with the ulcer personality tend to migrate to those areas where the opportunity for success is greater. Thus, the southern agricultural community where opportunities are few will not retain many of those with this inborn desire to achieve success.

Discussion

The ulcer personality has been described in terms of drive, multiple attempts at achievement, emotional responsiveness, self-reliance, responsibility, usually normal heterosexual adjustments, independence and determination. The intensity and the wholeheartedness with which these people carry out their self-imposed tasks and strive towards realization of their ambitions cannot be overemphasized. It is our belief that this intensive drive and the tension it creates as well as the inborn craving for superiority together with the worries generated by small failures, particularly the anxiety resulting from anticipated failure or future insecurity, are the emotional patterns which are fundamental in the production of ulcer.

Less than five minutes of questioning can determine the presence or absence of the typical ulcer personality. These patients are not difficult to question; in fact they are usually anxious to help. Unless the qualities mentioned in the preceding discussion are present in appreciable amounts, with not more than one significant exception, the patient is considered not to have a typical ulcer personality and questioning is directed toward other etiologic factors. Is there evidence of a neurosis, particularly with repressed dependent desires (Group B)? Has there been some unusually severe external precipitating situation (Group C)? Are constitutional, traumatic or x factors present in unusual degree (Group D)?

6

The Craving for Superiority

I T IS difficult to conceive that such a powerful force as the tremendous drive so characteristic of the typical ulcer personality could be generated by repressed dependent desires or could result from a distorted, repressed urge to suckle at the mother's breast. It seems more plausible that this drive is a positive factor, a primordial urge for success. The psychologic principles of Adler seem more applicable here than those of Freud.

The source of the drive in patients with peptic ulcer can perhaps best be understood in the light of the highly instructive monograph of Dodge and Kahn (16) entitled, *The Craving for Superiority*. They believed that the craving for superiority is one of the fundamental human traits, closely related to the instinct for self-preservation. They suggested that the survival of the fittest may be nothing more than Nature's stamp of approval on the overpowering importance and effect of superiority and on the craving for superiority she has created. They observed that one of the unusual characteristics of this craving for superiority is its insatiability. In this it resembles the craving to live with which it may be closely related. They pointed out that even in those with considerable real superiority there rarely appears any evidence of satiation, for great finan-

ciers and great scientists, like great generals, may sigh
for more worlds to conquer.

A person with a craving for superiority will attain
satisfactory goals of achievement provided he has the
equipment with which to achieve success and provided
he has set up reasonable goals. The person with a well
adjusted personality will set up real goals whereas the
neurotic person may set up false goals or he may even
be satisfied to strive for prestige instead of real accomplishment. Thus, one may speak of a person who has a
normal amount of desire for prestige but who is actually
motivated by a desire for real accomplishment
("healthy ambition"). He is conscious of the fact that
he lives and works for the environment. For him life is a
matter of achieving goals which consist of genuine
values. His antithesis is the individual who is ambitious
chiefly for prestige and who acts as though the world
existed for him alone. He strives not to serve humanity
but only to enhance his own prestige. For him it is a
matter of appearance, of pseudo values and goals. For
him the environment is not a field for genuine effort
but only a sounding board for his ego-prestige, a stage
for his vanity. For the person who is ambitious for accomplishment everything he seeks is genuine whereas
the person who is ambitious for prestige has no real goal.

Close observation for many years of patients with
peptic ulcer has strengthened our belief that the typical
ulcer personality is characterized by an insatiable craving for real superiority. It is perhaps fair to estimate that
approximately 10 or 15 per cent of people have any one
human trait in high degree, another 10 or 15 per cent
exhibit the same trait in low degree and 70 or 80 per
cent have an average amount of it. This is true for such

attributes as physical endurance, strength and intelligence, and the craving for superiority probably has a similar distribution. Many of the traits of the ulcer personality are common ones and the ulcer personality itself is probably one of the most common general types. Various surveys have indicated that from 10 to 12 per cent of the population suffer from peptic ulcer at some time in their lives and it is our belief that the distribution of the craving for superiority and the incidence of peptic ulcer are fairly closely related.

The strong craving for superiority in the patient with the typical ulcer personality is a real one; his values are genuine and any prestige which he gains in achieving them is of secondary importance. He is destined for a life of intense effort at attaining success and real matter-of-fact superiority through genuine achievement. Although healthy in direction, his ambition is almost pathologic in its intensity. The craving for accomplishment is practically insatiable at least during the most active decades of adult life. Satiability seems to be reached in most only in the sixth or seventh decade. No wonder patients with peptic ulcer drive themselves as they do; no wonder they are subjected to anxiety, tension, frustration and resentment at the obstacles in their path during a lifetime in which their goals are always ahead of them but never attained.

Dodge and Kahn clearly showed the perversions which may occur in this instinctive craving for superiority. They noted that certain persons accept as a substitute a *feeling of superiority* for *matter-of-fact* superiority and that in certain instances some even substitute an apparent *craving* for a *feeling of inferiority*. Patients with peptic ulcer crave a true *matter-of-*

fact superiority which they are determined to achieve whereas patients with ulcerative colitis, for example, are willing to settle for a *feeling* of superiority. Lacking a true superiority they set up pseudo values and goals and settle for a perversion of the real thing.

7

The Precipitating Situation

THE discussion thus far has dealt largely with the intrinsic emotional factors (originating within the personality) leading to peptic ulcer. The extrinsic emotional factors, those arising in the environment, cannot be completely separated from those arising from within. However, in the treatment of peptic ulcer it is advisable to recognize that sometimes it is easier to modify the environment than the personality or vice versa. So close is the relationship between personality and environment that we were tempted in our original formula to replace $b + c$ by $b \times c$, because if the ulcer personality is strong, the precipitating situation may be a minor one, and if the ulcer personality is absent, the precipitating situation may need to be strong. Often, peptic ulcer is the result of the product of the two factors and not their sum. Of course, this is not always true because a recurrence which would be brought on by a minor event would also be precipitated by a major catastrophe. For this reason the simpler formula was used.

Because of this variation in intensity it may be simpler to discuss the precipitating emotional situation in relation to the three personality types: the typical ulcer personality (Group A); the more neurotic (Group B); and the previously "normal" personality (Group C). Although emphasis is being placed on the emotional aspects of precipitating situations, this is not to deny that other factors such as respiratory infections, irritating oral medications or dietary indiscretions are occasionally responsible for recurrences. As long ago as 1935 Emery and Monroe (21) closely followed a group of patients with ulcer in an effort to determine the reason for relapses. They were impressed by the frequency with which three factors (fatigue, emotion and infection) seemed responsible. Fatigue preceded a relapse in 334 of 1,279 patients; emotional excitement was the reason for recurrence in 258 cases; infections, particularly of the upper respiratory tract, were responsible in 167 cases; and only 37 patients believed that indiscretions in diet were the cause.

Group A

The events which precipitate recurrences in patients with the typical ulcer personality usually are minor crises often related to the patient's occupation. For example, we have noted for many years that an auditor tends to have recurrences at the time of the year when he is under the greatest occupational stress and strain, that is toward the end of the fiscal year or when income tax reports are being prepared. During this time instead of eight hours he has to work ten or twelve hours a day at the office and frequently several more hours at night. Even if he did not work at night, he would be unable to relax in the evening and would awaken at night to find figures running through his head. After two or three weeks, the patient would find himself getting more and more wound up and less able to relax. He would be unable to get to sleep at night because of worry, he would awaken a number of times during the night when he finally did fall asleep, or he would awaken because of nightmares and be unable to go back to sleep. This would result in mild or moderately severe anxiety. Of course, this emotional tension would not be the only reason for recurrences. Of some importance are the extra five or ten cups of coffee or other stimulants which he would take to keep going, the increased consumption of tobacco and the irregular dietary habits.

The importance of the external precipitating situation in Group A has been demonstrated by the studies of Davies and Wilson (15). In 84 per cent of 205 cases of peptic ulcer the symptoms began soon, usually within five to seven days, after some event affecting the patient's work or finances or the health of his family. Only 22 of the 100 patients with hernia gave a history of any similar events preceding their illness. Of 52 relapses of peptic ulcer with craters proved by radiography, 42 were shown to have followed within three to five days some event causing anxiety. In most of their patients the anxiety was related to money matters, job security, increased responsibility at work, the possibility of dismissal or the illness or sudden death of a near relative. Davies and Wilson pointed out that in the patient with ulcer there is both the soil and the seed. The soil is represented by the tense, active person concerned more with external circumstances than with his own health whereas the seed is the acute anxiety which results from some reversal in fortune or some increased responsibility. The patient then begins to suffer from dyspepsia or rather from hunger pains, but if he eats regularly and frequently he may quickly obtain relief. If, however, he becomes engrossed in his work more deeply than usual because of his anxiety and goes long hours without food, an ulcer may develop. With attention to frequent feedings and medication the ulcer may heal and the symptoms disappear. The patient remains well until another emotional upset brings about a return of symptoms. Although most of their patients were people of small means who depended for their well-being on the money they earned each week, they noted no difference in their private practices where anxieties were over matters of larger dimension.

It has already been pointed out that these people are extremely active, hard working individuals who always drive themselves at close to top speed every day. When an emergency arises, they will draw on their remaining energy, but if the crisis is too severe and too prolonged or if a succession of minor crises occurs, they will reach their limit of endurance. They become more and more tense and anxious but keep trying to spur their mind and body to further accomplishments; they do not voluntarily quit. As we know from the investigations of Wolf and Wolff (52), this is the type of emotional reaction which results in gastric hyperfunction. This continued hyperfunction is probably the most important contributing factor in ulcer recurrence.

Wolf and Wolff (52) pointed out that the principal difference between the emotional reactions accompanying gastric hyperfunction on one hand and hypofunction on the other appears to be whether or not the subject continues fighting or has given up. The individual whose stomach is hyperactive is physiologically prepared for food whether or not he has an appetite. If he is about to meet his situational threat, he feels the need of being fed or cared for. The individual who considers himself defeated and whose stomach is hypoactive is not accepting the challenge of the situational threat. His associated nausea expresses his distaste for the situation. Thus the stomach's reactions to adverse life situations which give rise to anxiety and conflict may express the way in which the organism proposes to deal with the problem.

We agree with Davies and Wilson that in most cases a return of ulcer symptoms follows only a few days after changes in work habits, financial difficulties or misfortune to some member of the family (Cases 2, 3) which thrust further responsibility on the patient. For example, in Kaufmann's case (28) previously cited the lawyer's hemorrhages were associated with prolonged court trials. Physicians interested in the treatment of peptic ulcer should take an interest in their patients' occupations and should try to learn the stresses and strains associated with the major types of occupation. If one is familiar with much of this information, it is relatively easy to determine any distressing situations which may have preceded the recurrence. It has been our experience that from 85 to 90 per cent of recurrences in Group A are preceded by relatively minor crises in the lives of the patients.

We have never been impressed by any significant increase in the incidence of recurrences during the spring or fall. Numerous instances in which the patient himself has mentioned that he had recurrences in the spring or fall have been traced to occupational hazards or increased responsibilities during these seasons of the year. Zane (53) also believes that recurrences are due to the patient's seasonal problems rather than to the time of year. Those interested in this factor are referred to the excellent discussion of Palmer (37).

Group B

In the more neurotic group, the precipitating situation is usually more complex, that is, more involved with their neurotic life entanglements. The precipitating event is usually more dramatic and intense but this may not be appreciated unless the emotional conflict is uncovered (Cases 5, 7–9). The first interview will rarely uncover the basis of the deep-seated neurosis and therefore the nature of the precipitating circumstance may not be appreciated. In this unraveling of the relation between the onset of symptoms and the complexities of the interpersonal situation, the psychiatrist is indispensable. Recurrences in this group may be associated with episodes in the patient's other psychosomatic disorders such as asthma, hyperventilation syndrome, hypertension or rheumatism.

Group C

To paraphrase the old proverb, some men are born to have ulcers (Group A), some acquire ulcers (Group B), and others have ulcers thrust upon them (Group C). According to our observations those in Group C with previously normal personalities are the ones who have thrust upon them from the outside world some unusually severe, emotionally upsetting situation which gives rise to an anxiety state, usually acute and of relatively short duration. Because of the intensity of the precipitating situation and the severity of the induced anxiety, an acute ulcer develops.

The incidence of ulcers is strikingly influenced by the amount of anxiety and tension in the international and domestic situations. Depressions, wars and similar ex-

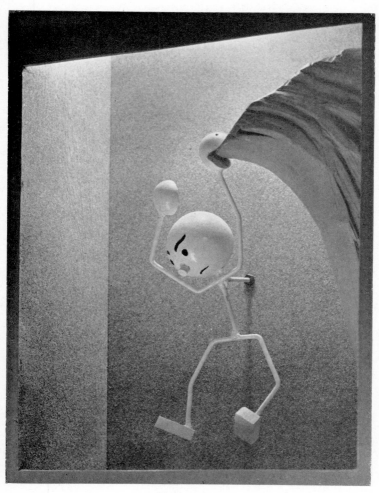

FIGURE 10

INSECURE

periences have always briefly and temporarily increased
the number of such cases. For example, in the first five
days following the attack on Pearl Harbor on Dec. 7,
1941, one of us saw three cases of perforated peptic
ulcer in men in the sixth decade of life who had had no
previous ulcer symptoms and who were apparently
perfectly normal. All three perforations occurred at
night and all three patients admitted that beginning
with December seventh they had lain awake each night
worrying about sons in the Armed Forces stationed in
the Pacific area. All felt the frustration of being "unable
to do anything about it." We have not seen three cases
of perforated ulcer in persons of that age with no previous ulcer symptoms in any five-year period before or
since.

These are probably the cases referred to by Davies
and Wilson (15) when they wrote, "In some the dyspepsia and ulcer formation occurred for the first time
at the mature age of 60 but in such cases, as a rule, the
event preceding the symptoms was outstanding." These
are the patients with hemorrhage or acute perforation
brought into the hospitals of England during the blitz
along with the bomb casualties (39). Stewart and
Winser (46) observed that during the severest blitz
months, September and October 1940, the number of
patients with perforated ulcers admitted to 16 London
hospitals rose from a previous average of 23 a month to
64. Melton (33) noticed a similar rise in cases of hematemesis at the outbreak of World War II in September
1939. These are the New York brokers in whom symptoms developed about a week after the stock market
crash in October 1929. These are the individuals all over
the country without previous ulcer symptoms in whom

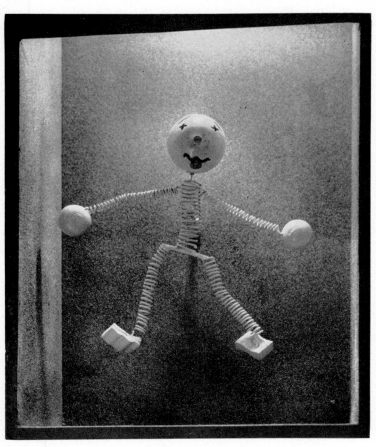

FIGURE 11

DISSONANT

ulcers developed for the first time when their banks closed or the mortgages were foreclosed on their homes during the black days of the economic depression of 1929 to 1932. These are the people who have been thrust into an acute anxiety state by some overwhelming situation (Cases 10–12).

Since the precipitating situation itself may be self-limited and nonrecurring, the recognition of cases which fall in Group C has great diagnostic, prognostic and therapeutic significance. Many cases of hematemesis of "unknown etiology" probably fall into this category. Such patients may well have acute erosions which heal promptly and are not seen gastroscopically or roentgenographically when studied a week or two later.

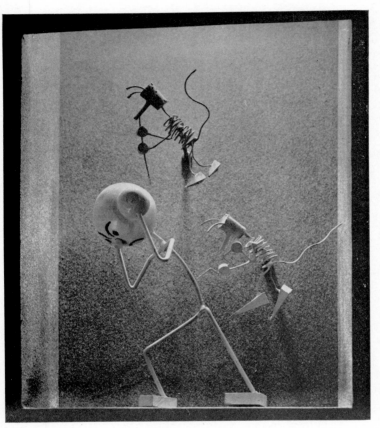

FIGURE 12

DRIVEN

8

Inter-relation of Various Etiologic Factors

THE relative importance of the various etiologic factors in peptic ulcer have been discussed in considerable detail. This has been summarized in Table II. A hypothesis to explain the inter-relation of the various etiologic factors based on this outline will now be offered.

Both the craving for superiority and the craving for affection are fundamental human traits with the usual distribution curve. In order to produce an ulcer on a psychosomatic basis it is necessary for a person to have more than the median amount of both of these characteristics. At the same time, it is possible that more than the median amount of genetic, constitutional, traumatic and x factors is required to supplement the emotional factors. Certainly no amount of a, b, c and d factors will ordinarily produce an ulcer in the absence of hydrochloric acid in the stomach.

Figure 13 represents graphically the normal distribution curve for any human trait (29), drawn according to an arbitrary scale of 4 — to 4 + with a median of 0. On the basis of this scale some of the blanks in Table II can be assigned values. The result, Table III, is, like any other hypothesis, subject to revision but we believe it supplies the best answers available to the questions posed by Dunbar (20), who thinks that in order to

DISTRIBUTION CURVE OF ANY HUMAN TRAIT

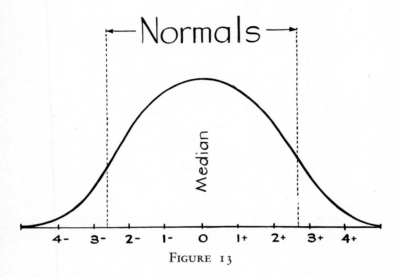

FIGURE 13

understand any psychosomatic illness three questions must be answered. (1) What is it in a personality which generates the predisposition to illness? (2) What determines the choice of the specific expression of the illness? (3) What is the precipitating factor which brings on the illness?

In Group A the anxiety-tension state resulting from the inability to satisfy an insatiable hunger for real superiority predisposes to the illness. It expresses itself in the stomach rather than the heart or lungs because of an above median, but still normal, amount of craving for affection (they feel with their stomachs) plus a combination of *a, d* and *x* factors. The precipitating

TABLE I

LIABILITY TO PEPTIC ULCER

Age	Percentage Danger Past
Under 20	0
20–24	3
25–29	8
30–34	22
35–39	40
40–44	57
45–49	72
50–54	82
55–59	91
60–64	94
65–69	97
70–74	99
Over 75	100

factors of the recurrent episodes are usually related to job, money or illness, which threaten to frustrate the desire for success.

In Group B are those dissonant personalities who by the intensity of their conflicts are driven into illness. The stomach is the "shock organ" because, as shown by Alexander, it is intimately bound up with their neurosis by the repression of their oral receptive tendencies. The precipitating factor is usually a crisis in interpersonal relations.

In Group C are those with high ideals who are often perfectionists and have more than a median (but still normal) amount of craving for affection. There is not enough internal combustion generated from these two factors to produce an ulcer, but the spark is there and when a calamity strikes, the flame is ignited. If these persons did not have more than the median craving for superiority and affection, the external precipitating

TABLE II

RELATIVE IMPORTANCE OF ETIOLOGIC FACTORS IN PEPTIC ULCER

Group	Craving for Superiority	Craving for Love and Affection (repressed)	Intensity of the Precipitating Situation	Intensity of Constitutional, Traumatic and x Factors
A Ulcer Personality	4 +		1 or 2 +	
B Neurotic Personality		4 +	2 or 3 +	
C Anxiety States			4 +	
D No Personality Deviation				4 +

TABLE III

NUMERICAL SUMMATION OF ETIOLOGIC FACTORS
IN PEPTIC ULCER

Group	Craving for Superiority	Craving for Love and Affection	Intensity of the Precipitating Situation	Intensity of Constitutional, Traumatic and x Factors
A	4 +	1 or 2 +	1 or 2 +	1 or 2 +
B	1 or 2 +	4 +	2 or 3 +	1 or 2 +
C	1 or 2 +	1 or 2 +	4 +	1 or 2 +
D	0	0	0	4 +

situation would have resulted not in an ulcer but in some other psychosomatic manifestation such as migraine, asthma or hypertension because of other ways of experiencing events.

The emotional response common to Groups A, B and C seems to be anxiety and, although it is usually variously associated with frustration, resentment, hostility and guilt, we must again marvel at the perspicuity of Brinton, who stated ninety years ago that "we are fully entitled to regard it [anxiety] as a more or less immediate cause" of ulcer.

Comment

We have entered into the field of psychology and psychiatry with some temerity. We realize that there is nothing so intricate and difficult to describe as the human personality. We often forget that mankind is a curious mixture of good and evil, of strength and weakness, of love and hate and that some dependence as well as independence on affection are present in all of us. Ambivalence and ambitendence are universal traits. But all these traits we describe so glibly are each in themselves a complicated amalgamation of components none of which can actually be measured. Each of us tends to find the things that we seek and in which we are interested. Our reactions to a given patient will vary with our own personalities. The physician instinctively likes one patient and dislikes the next one he sees at least partially on the basis of his own personal reaction to certain prominent traits in the patient and in himself.

We believe that too much is being written on the emotional factors in peptic ulcer by those who have seen but a relatively small number of ulcer patients and often these are of selected groups seen only in a mental institution, a charity hospital (31) or in an institution with large numbers of alcoholic patients. The psychiatrist who interviews such a restricted group of poorly selected patients naturally finds a higher percentage of failures and of frustrated neurotic personalities.

9

Observations and Predictions

THERE are certain clinical features of the ulcer problem which are of interest. First, since Group A is by far the largest group, it may be designated the most typical. Thus, as would be expected, it contains the highest percentage of the textbook type of ulcer, that is, the chronic duodenal ulcer of twenty years' duration with its frequent recurrences. A smaller percentage of women would be expected in this group since ulcer is predominantly a male disease. In a recent report (47) of a small series of active ulcers the ratio of males to females in Group A was 35 to one and in all other groups combined was eight to seven.

Since Group B is by definition the neurotic group, one would expect to find in it most of the patients with other neurotic manifestations and other psychosomatic syndromes—those whose symptoms are bizarre and out of proportion to the clinical findings, the alcoholic addict, those with manic-depressive swings and most, but not all, women with peptic ulcer. This has been our experience.

In Group C we would expect and do find most of the cases of acute ulcer. More than 70 per cent of the "silent" ulcers which bleed or perforate without previous warning fall in this group, small as it is.

In Group D will fall most ulcers associated with

epigastric or hiatal hernias, with bezoars and with the other more unusual causes as illustrated by Cases 13–17. Here too will be the cases of ulcer developing in a Meckel's diverticulum and the anastomotic ulcers which develop after gastroenterostomy for initial lesions other than peptic ulcer.

These observations are of value, particularly in the appraisal of various forms of therapy. The ultimate worth of any new form of medical treatment can best be determined in typical cases (Group A). For example, since this group is so predominantly male, the evaluation of a new form of therapy based on a group of patients, 31 per cent of whom are females (23), will be misleading. Such a group will contain a high percentage of atypical cases with many more acute, nonrecurring ulcers than are to be expected on a chance basis. Results obtained in such cases are naturally better than average and cannot be ascribed solely to treatment.

Evaluation of the newer surgical procedures for "cure" of ulcers should also be based on cases in Group A. Patients in Group C rarely need surgical treatment other than emergency surgical procedures for perforation or occasionally for prolonged hemorrhage. It has already been pointed out (35) that vagotomy for a patient who has a peptic ulcer associated with a deep-seated neurosis does not cure the neurosis, and many neurotic gastrointestinal symptoms may persist after the operation. In our recent experience most cases of the dumping syndrome following subtotal gastrectomy have been patients with neuroses (Group B).

10

Treatment

I⊤ is not the purpose of this monograph to elaborate on the treatment of peptic ulcer except to emphasize that adequate treatment depends upon proper evaluation of the numerous etiologic factors involved in the production of each individual case of peptic ulcer. If constitutional factors are present, there is no question that the prophylactic treatment designed to prevent the development of ulcers is important. Dietary restrictions, particularly at times of stress and strain, prompt attention to even the normal amount of dyspepsia and avoidance of internal and external trauma are all indicated.

Recognition that the external precipitating emotional situations are particularly concerned with the patient's occupation has been, in our experience, the most important single measure in the prevention of recurrences. The occupational tensions can usually be predicted and measures can thus be instituted to prevent recurrences. We prescribe antispasmodics, antacids, sedatives and special diets, as do most gastroenterologists, to modify d and x factors, but we try to employ them in the prevention of recurrences as well as in the treatment of active cases of ulcer. By giving the patients a thorough understanding of the importance of these precipitating factors, we are able to guide them into intelligent use of these prophylactic measures so that they are able to prevent about 80 per cent of predicted recurrences.

To illustrate, the case of the auditor may again be cited. When the period of the year approaches during which he is to be under the greatest stress, he should be instructed to adhere strictly to a special diet for ulcer with frequent feedings between meals. He should take an antispasmodic and an antacid regularly and a mild sedative occasionally. By the use of these measures throughout this period of increased stresses and strains he will usually be able to avoid recurrences.

It has been our experience that patients with the typical ulcer personality are intolerant of psychiatrists just as they are of their diets, their stomach and anything else which impedes their activity. Occasionally, they may consult a psychiatrist when advised to do so but as soon as their symptoms subside they will fail to return. All patients in Group B (those with a pronounced tendency to deep-seated neuroses) need psychiatric care. Although their ulcers may be handled successfully without psychotherapy, recurrences are common, and to manage the whole problem successfully psychiatric aid is needed. In Group C the acute precipitating situation may be self limited and may clear up without psychiatric assistance, for the patient may be able to understand his anxiety and thus cope with the situation alone; occasionally the anxiety may be so severe as to require psychotherapy.

It has been our observation over a period of years that from 10 to 15 per cent of patients with peptic ulcer will greatly benefit from psychiatric treatment but only 2 to 3 per cent will seek psychiatric acid. Consequently, the gastroenterologist or the internist must supply most of the necessary psychotherapy; in fact only he can give advice to the patients in Group A (typical ulcer personality). The patient comes to the physician because of abdominal pain. If to abolish this pain it is necessary to modify his habits, the physician can best convince the patient of this necessity and can best work out the details of how it is to be done. Such advice will be accepted from the physician who is honest enough to tell his patient that unless he alters his way of living, he is bound to have recurrences. To obtain the best results the physician must have a thorough understanding of the disease and the personality in which it occurs and he must be able to show the patient why these modifications in the craving for superiority are necessary. This must be done with wisdom and understanding and not by thoughtlessly proscribing all activity and leaving the patient more miserable than before. It is often advisable to point out to the patient that he can do perhaps as much and certainly a better quality of work if he will take long week ends away from his work, go on adequate annual vacations, make an effort to secure some regular exercise as an outlet for his energy and particularly make continued efforts to modify his drive.

In conclusion, it has been our experience that the most frequent error on the part of physicians in the handling of patients with peptic ulcer is to ascribe all ulcers to some single pet etiologic agent, and consequently to become attached to one form of therapy to the exclusion of all others. Brown (10), who has frequently warned against this tendency, aptly paraphrased Pope when he wrote:

Each champion, to the other's virtue blind
And thinks *his* treatment only cures mankind.

11

Report of Cases

THE following are examples of cases with the typical ulcer personality (Group A); intrinsic neurotic conflicts (Group B); pronounced environmental stresses (Group C) and other etiologic factors (Group D).

Group A

Case 1: N.D., a 44-year-old business man, who looked ten years older, consulted us because of dyspepsia of fifteen years' duration. He had the ulcer habitus. He was slender, of medium height with a narrow costal angle, a scaphoid abdomen, dilated pupils, overactive knee jerks, cold sweaty palms and feet and a blood pressure of 105 diastolic and 65 systolic. He also had the typical ulcer personality. He had been married twenty years but had never been on a vacation since his honeymoon. He had never been away from home for more than two or three days at a time and then only on business. In addition to owning and operating several retail gasoline stations, he was a wholesale gasoline and oil distributor, he had a separate wholesale automobile parts business and owned and operated a small coal mine. Since the end of World War II he had been engaged in building homes and service stations in various parts of his state, usually having three or four in the process of construction at one time. He held an office in practically every civic and political organization in his county and was an active religious worker.

He had had abdominal pain for fifteen years, but five months before we saw him, the pain had radiated to his back and was so severe that he consulted a physician for the first time. He was subjected to great emotional strain at that time because his only daughter had left her husband and returned with her two small children to live with him. Our studies revealed a deformity of the duodenal cap secondary to cicatricial changes of a chronic duodenal ulcer.

Comment: This case is characteristic of the patient with a typical ulcer in nearly every respect. He had the ulcer habitus; there was a long history of the dyspepsia characteristic of peptic ulcer for which he did not consult a physician for nearly fifteen years. He worked long hours without a day off for twenty-seven years. When his daughter's marriage dissolved, his symptoms became more severe and he was forced to seek medical attention.

Case 2: C.W., a 40-year-old housewife, gave a typical history of duodenal ulcer with positive roentgenographic findings. Her symptoms began at the age of 18 when she was a senior high school student in charge of a school carnival and "doing 90 per cent of the work and 100 per cent of the worrying about it." For one week she had been working at top speed every day and until late at night in preparation for the event. She was on her way to the carnival when she suddenly felt weak, broke out in a sweat, became nauseated and vomited dark red blood. She vomited four more times during the night, had tarry stools for two days and was hospitalized. A month later she was operated on for appendicitis but the appendix was found to be normal. She had no further difficulty until the depths of the economic depression about ten years later. At that time she had been married seven years and had two young children. The bank failed, leaving them financially embarrassed and for the first time the patient began to have typical ulcer symptoms of periodic epigastric pain relieved by food. Because these symptoms persisted, a roentgenogram of her stomach was made which revealed a duodenal ulcer. Dietary measures gave relief until four years ago. At that time her father became ill and in addition to her own duties she assumed the responsibility of managing his dairy farm as well as his household. The patient's mother was hospitalized during this period and while visiting her one day the patient again had a hemorrhage and fainted. She was kept in bed for four months and felt well until September 1945 when her husband had an attack of coronary occlusion and the patient had to manage his contracting business for six months. During this time her epigastric pain recurred. Again she began to get weak and noticed tarry stools for about two weeks. She was hospitalized and put on a strict ulcer regimen once more. Shortly before we saw her, her mother broke her hip, and the patient's responsibilities again increased and her symptoms recurred.

The patient's personality is best described in her own words, "Whenever I join an organization I soon find myself being made president or secretary and doing practically all the work." All during her married life she had assumed many civic responsibilities. Just before she came to the Ochsner Clinic, in spite of her symptoms and her mother's illness, she had been running a hot dog and soft drink concession several nights a week at a local baseball park in order to raise funds for a woman's club.

Comment: This is an example of a person with a long-standing duodenal ulcer who has the typical ulcer personality and in whom the precipitating situations have always been the ordinary events such as increased responsibilities, financial difficulties or family misfortunes.

Case 3: R.J., a 39-year-old minister, had typical ulcer discomfort for thirty-three years, beginning at the age of six when he first started working on his father's farm. The patient's mother and his only brother also had duodenal ulcers. The patient had the typical ulcer constitution and also the ulcer personality. Although he was full time minister, he took a full time job in the ship yards during the war not primarily because of the money but rather because he wanted to be of service. When we saw him in 1947, he was studying for an advanced degree at a college more than 300 miles from his pastorate and was carrying a heavy schedule. He would finish his studies on Saturday noon, write his sermon while traveling the 300 miles home and then spend all Saturday night and Sunday with his church members, visiting the sick, attending board meetings and conducting services. Then he would have to spend all Sunday night traveling 300 miles to attend class on Monday morning.

Comment: This case presents a poor genetic background, a typical ulcer constitution and a typical ulcer personality.

Case 4: F.E., a 47-year-old married woman, came to the Ochsner Clinic because of a recent gastrointestinal hemorrhage. Her symptoms began approximately at the age of 20 years when she was earning her own living as a physiotherapist and was studying for an advanced degree. A few years later she married and her symptoms disappeared for nearly a year. Then her husband had to be hospitalized because of tuberculosis and it was necessary for her to work to support herself and pay his sanatorium bills. Within the next year her symptoms recurred, and continued for the next four years at the end of which time her husband died. For the next two years, although she supported herself, her symptoms were less severe. Ten years ago she remarried, and her symptoms entirely disappeared. Three months before we saw her, her husband suffered an attack of coronary occlusion, followed by an anxiety-depression with a complete change in personality. Although for ten years they had been completely congenial, since his illness her husband became exceedingly irritable and was afraid to partake in any of his previous activities or interests because of his doctor's warning. While under this strain and preparing Christmas festivities for her two young children, the patient had a sudden hemorrhage.

Comment: This is an example of the typical ulcer personality as seen in some women. The patient was a good mixer, accepted many social, civic and religious responsibilities, was a good business woman and always had been able to take care of herself and her family if necessary. The remission during the first ten years of a happy second marriage is rather typical.

Group B

Case 5: B.L., a 37-year-old boiler tender, had had periodic epigastric discomfort typical of peptic ulcer for ten years. Our studies revealed an active duodenal ulcer.

He had few if any of the characteristic traits of the ulcer personality but he was suffering from a severe chronic anxiety state. He had extreme claustrophobia and had a deadly fear of having to climb into a boiler, which unfortunately was a necessary part of his job from time to time. The mere suggestion that he might have to get inside of the boiler to do some repairs would cause him to have nightmares or insomnia and would always bring on a recurrence of the ulcer symptoms. In addition, he had a cancer phobia which developed after an aunt died from cancer of the stomach. For many years he had been working on one shift but during the past four months it was necessary for him to change shifts every seven days. This had so upset his daily routine that continuous gastric symptoms resulted. Because of his severe chronic anxiety state we doubted that he would respond to a medical regimen of antispasmodics, sedatives, diet and psychotherapy. However, three months after his discharge he wrote that he had gained 30 pounds and that his symptoms had not recurred. Despite this improvement we do not believe that the ultimate prognosis with medical treatment is good.

Comment: This is an example of an ulcer developing in a patient with a deep-seated neurosis who had none of the characteristics of the typical ulcer personality.

Case 6: B.B., a 61-year-old business man, had never had any previous significant gastrointestinal symptoms. Five months before he consulted us in 1945 coronary thrombosis developed. He was kept in bed for twelve weeks and told that he must sell his business interest and never work again. Largely because of the pessimism of his physician he became extremely anxious and agitated. He sold his business interest to his brother and then became concerned for fear that he had exacted too high a price. He became depressed, would recognize no one but his wife and would not leave his bed although bed rest was no longer required. Six electric shock treatments resulted in slight temporary improvement, but his anxiety and depression again became severe. During this period he complained of some epigastric pain relieved by milk or soda and several weeks before coming to the Clinic he had tarry stools for five days. A roentgenogram at that time disclosed a duodenal ulcer. A roentgenogram taken after we saw him revealed a duodenal ulcer with a crater. This patient did not have the typical ulcer personality but certainly was suffering from a severe acute anxiety state. Treatment consisted of the usual ulcer regimen, the use of sedatives at night and dextro-amphetamine sulfate in the morning and one psychotherapeutic session. His anxiety state and depression promptly disappeared. He has been followed for two years, has gained 40 pounds and has had no recurrence of the epigastric distress. Today he is a happy, well-adjusted individual and lives an unrestricted life.

Comment: This ulcer, due to an acute anxiety state, may be classified in Group B. The acute precipitating situation was the attack of coronary occlusion.

Case 7: M.J., a 32-year-old white housewife, had symptoms of peptic ulcer for eight years. Symptoms characteristic of a duodenal ulcer first appeared during a severe attack of Brill's disease, which lasted for some weeks. A roentgenogram at that time is said to have confirmed the diagnosis of duodenal ulcer. Medical treatment was not successful and partial gastrectomy performed about four years before we saw the patient provided relief for a year or two, but then symptoms recurred. For a year before the patient consulted us she had almost continuous pain and considerable vomiting and had lost about 20 pounds.

When we first saw her, she appeared to have none of the characteristic ulcer personality traits and denied any emotional upsets. A jejunal ulcer was suspected; a crater could never be demonstrated although there was some narrowing of the afferent loop. Medical treatment in the hospital relieved none of the symptoms but the vomiting. The patient was sent home with instructions to follow a strict medical regimen; in six months she returned begging for another operation because of continuous symptoms. At subtotal gastrectomy, some slight scarring and kinking of the afferent loop of the gastroenterostomy could be seen but there was no active ulcer crater. For approximately three months postoperatively she gained weight and felt well but then had a recurrence of vomiting and pain. These symptoms were exactly the same as she had the year before and a psychiatric consultation quickly revealed the difficulty.

The symptoms for which the patient consulted us had occurred immediately after the following episode. The patient's mother had intestinal obstruction and congestive heart failure and the patient was told that her mother would die if she was not operated upon but that because of her cardiac condition, she would probably die if she was. After consulting other members of the family the patient gave her permission for the operation; the mother died on the operating table. The patient herself had a strong feeling of guilt about this and it was enhanced by relatives who blamed her for making the decision which killed her mother. The epigastric pain and vomiting began immediately and were relieved only after subtotal gastrectomy. She had no further trouble until the following episode three months later. She was taking care of her sister who was in the hospital following the birth of a child. About the fourth or fifth postpartum day the patient relieved her brother-in-law of his bedside vigil late in the evening. Because of recent lack of sleep she dozed off for a few minutes and awoke to find her sister dead. Again a severe guilt reaction developed. She believed that if she had not dozed off, her sister would not have died. Considerable improvement followed a few psychotherapeutic sessions. The patient has had no recurrences.

Comment: This is an example of an ulcer in a neurotic person with an obvious guilt reaction. It also illustrates how difficult it is to determine the acute precipitating situation in some instances. This patient repeatedly denied emotional upsets to us but the psychiatrist uncovered the neurosis in one interview.

Case 8: S.R., a 45-year-old professional man, consulted us because of an active duodenal ulcer. He was engaged in many outside business activities and had assumed a number of civic responsibilities. He did not have the usual ulcer personality; he was deliberate in many of his mannerisms and in his way of talking and thinking. In childhood and during college he showed no evidence of an ulcer personality. Unfortunately, he married a woman with many psychopathic traits. His successful professional career is largely the result of his unhappy domestic life; it has been an escape and a reason for him to be away from home the maximum amount of time. No doubt his accomplishments have been a substitute for affection.

His gastric symptoms began five months before we saw him on the very day he finally decided to seek a divorce after considering it for a year or more. Divorce was sought only after he obtained psychiatric advice concerning its effect on the children. All this time he was under tremendous tension because of his wife's behavior. She first agreed to the divorce but changed her mind repeatedly and until the day the divorce was granted he was never sure that she would allow it to go through. It is interesting that his ulcer symptoms ceased on the day the divorce was granted.

Comment: This patient was thrust into his numerous activities by an intolerable domestic situation. His ulcer was the result of a combination of many years of domestic tension and the uncertainty of his divorce proceedings. The mechanism is typical of that described by Alexander.

Case 9: F.R., a 38-year-old housewife, came to the Ochsner Clinic because of intestinal parasites (enterobius vermicularis) and for a check up of an old duodenal ulcer. She was a happily married housewife whose ulcer symptoms began at the age of 18 years. We could find no evidence of the usual ulcer personality, there were no severe acute precipitating episodes in her life and there was no family background of ulcer. The patient had a slight speech defect and when asked if she was left handed related that although she was naturally left handed her father insisted she do things with her right hand. She has vivid recollections of a childhood in which she was constantly being corrected for using her left hand. A speech defect and certain other mannerisms developed along with a slight facial tic and she was never able to write a good hand. Although she never learned to feel at ease with people because of her speech defect, she took a secretarial course and at the age of 18 years accepted a secretarial position in a busy office where it was necessary for her to meet people continually. It was during this trying period that her ulcer symptoms began. Since her marriage she has had few gastric symptoms.

Comment: It is our belief that the ulcer symptoms in this case were almost entirely due to personality deviations and were precipitated by a job requiring her to work under such trying circumstances. The precipitating situation would have been a relatively minor experience to most 18-year-old girls, but it was significant in this case because of the patient's neurotic way of experiencing new personal contacts.

Group C

Case 10: G.E., a 53-year-old ship's carpenter, consulted us in August 1945 because of severe and continuous gastric symptoms of eight months' duration. At an early age the patient's seafaring parents were lost running guns to the revolutionists in Cuba prior to the Spanish-American War. Although he was a steady, conscientious workman with an excellent reputation among sea captains, he did not have the usual ulcer personality. He had none of the drive of the ulcer personality; in fact, since maritime pay had been so high he remained ashore for three or four months at a time just

"to take things easy." He never experienced any gastrointestinal symptoms until after the second ship was
torpedoed from under him in 1942 although his war
experiences up to that time had been severe and continuous since being bombed in the Suez Canal in the
latter part of 1939. Most of this period he spent either
in the North Atlantic or in the Mediterranean. Following his rescue from the second torpedoing, he was hospitalized. Because of his recent digestive complaints
roentgenograms were made, and these led to a diagnosis
of duodenal ulcer. After six weeks of treatment he returned to sea and was actively engaged in the North
African, Sicilian and Italian invasions. Although he lost
another one of his ships at Anzio, his symptoms did not
recur and he did well until December, 1944. At that
time he spent 36 continuous days at Antwerp when it
was under continuous and terrific bombardment. During this entire time he was unable to get any sleep other
than fifteen or twenty minute catnaps and he was under
constant terrifying strain as he daily watched many of
the neighboring vessels and warehouses blown up and
many of his friends killed. After about ten days of this
his ulcer symptoms recurred and were severe and continuous until he consulted us.

When we saw him, he was suffering from a severe
anxiety state, with pronounced insomnia, a curious type
of rapid, shallow breathing and continuous epigastric
pain. He also had a severe "startle reaction" and gross
tremor of the tongue and hand. These symptoms sub-
sided after a month of heavy sedation and frequent
psychotherapeutic interviews. Since his severe gastric
symptoms had been continuous for nearly eight months,
we were not surprised to find considerable deformity of

the duodenum. His symptoms eventually cleared up but he has had one recurrence and may eventually require surgical treatment as we suspect penetration into the pancreas and it is difficult for him to follow a diet while at sea.

Comment: This is a case of an ulcer which developed in an essentially normal person who was subjected to great emotional strain as a merchant mariner during the war. The first ulcer symptoms occurred after his second torpedoing and recurred approximately two years later during the blitz on Antwerp. At the time we saw him, he was suffering from a severe anxiety state.

Case 11: D.J., a 70-year-old physician who enjoyed good health and who had had no prior digestive symptoms, suffered mild dyspepsia for a few days and then passed tarry stools for several days. Complete studies revealed an active duodenal ulcer.

He did not have the typical ulcer personality. Although a successful practitioner, he had managed to live a relatively calm life with ample time to enjoy his family and with a reasonable amount of relaxation and recreation. There were no obvious genetic or traumatic factors and no evidence of any deep neuroses. The patient had been living alone for several years since the death of his wife but remained in close contact with his married children and his numerous friends. His life was serene until a few months before the gastric episode when he began to be annoyed continually by a psychopathic female patient who would appear at his office and home at all hours and would even accost him on the street. Refusing to take legal action or have the woman committed, he decided to retire from practice, sell the old homestead and go to live with a daughter in another state. This meant severing the ties of a lifetime and was undertaken with considerable reluctance. The dyspepsia and hemorrhage occurred while he was in the process of closing his office. On the usual ulcer regimen he quickly regained his former health and has remained well for a year without dietary restrictions.

Comment: This case illustrates the remark of Davies and Wilson that when an ulcer occurs for the first time after the mature age of 60, the event preceding the symptoms is usually outstanding. The precipitating emotional event in this instance was of great magnitude to the patient. One would not ordinarily expect a recurrence unless the patient is subjected to another equally distressing situation.

Case 12: S.J., a 52-year-old wife of a farmer, had had a moderate amount of periodic indigestion for about five years. These attacks were invariably associated with anxiety over her husband's drinking bouts. She was not of the ulcer personality type. On July 5, 1946, approximately one month before we saw her, she had an attack of hematemesis and melena. On the night of July 3, the patient had to carry her drunken husband home when he became involved in a fight at a dance. The patient is devoutly religious and much opposed to drinking and was considerably upset over this incident. She was unable to sleep that night and the following day she felt "sick at my stomach, nauseated and unable to eat." Again on the night of July 4 she was sleepless and remembers thinking, "what makes it so bad is that there is nothing I can do about it because I couldn't possibly divorce him." The next morning she vomited blood and passed tarry stools. Our studies revealed a small crater in the duodenal cap.

Comment: This is an example of the acute precipitating external emotional situation resulting in repeated attacks of indigestion and eventually hemorrhage, each attack being directly related to the patient's husband's alcoholic sprees.

Group D

Case 13: F.T. had none of the personality traits characteristic of peptic ulcer. He had no ambition and had received charity for some years. He consulted us because of gastric symptoms of two weeks' duration with vomiting of blood. On the day of the hemorrhage the patient had partaken of a large amount of a concoction known as "smoke," which is made by adding water to shellac to precipitate out the resinous substances and pouring off the supernatant fluid (of a high alcoholic content). Three of seven men who had imbibed this concoction died that night. The patient vomited a great deal and eventually vomited a large amount of coffee-ground material. On the next day he passed some tarry stools. He visited the eye dispensary about a week later for some difficulty in vision which in the light of the history suggests the possibility of methyl alcohol poisoning. Roentgenograms at that time showed a characteristic gastric ulcer on the lesser curvature with the niche near the angulus. A strict Sippy regimen for eight weeks resulted in disappearance of the crater. This patient was followed for five years and had had no recurrence.

Comment: This case may be classified as a chemical or traumatic ulcer, since a gastric ulcer developed in this man who had never had any previous gastric symptoms, as the result of drinking a chemical concoction potent enough to kill three out of seven persons.

Case 14: C.J., a 37-year-old wife of a physician, did not have the ulcer personality and showed no evidence of any significant neurosis. She had never had any previous gastrointestinal symptoms. In September 1945 a severe, persistent attack of sinusitis occurred for the first time in her life. Treatment consisted of daily packs in both nostrils and the liberal use of naphazoline. Following several weeks of practically continuous medication with these nose drops she experienced epigastric pain approximately two hours after meals which was relieved by food or antacids. In December 1945 she noted tarry stools, and sudden hematemesis required transfusions. While in the hospital naphazoline was discontinued, a strict ulcer regimen was followed and, of course, all symptoms disappeared. After she returned home, she continued the ulcer diet but gastric symptoms recurred, presumably because of the resumption of the naphazoline medication. A roentgenogram revealed an active duodenal ulcer.

Comment: This is an example of an ulcer probably caused by the pharmacologic action (chiefly vasoconstriction) of large amounts of naphazoline.

Case 15: A.G., a 48-year-old single man, came to the Ochsner Clinic with persistent gastric complaints of one and one half years' duration. Although he worked twelve to fourteen hours a day for seven days a week as a recreation director, he had none of the other characteristics of the typical ulcer personality. His gastric symptoms began a few hours after eating six persimmons while on a hunting trip. He gave a history of the ingestion of persimmons occasionally since childhood. Roentgenologic examination revealed an ulcer on the lesser curvature of the stomach and a movable foreign body in its lumen measuring approximately 10 cm. by 6 cm. At operation both a phytobezoar and a benign gastric ulcer were observed.

Comment: This is an illustration of a traumatic ulcer resulting from the continuous irritation of a phytobezoar.

Case 16: S.F. had none of the characteristics of the ulcer personality, but rather was a typical professional jazz musician. Prior to 1938 he had had no history suggesting a peptic ulcer. In 1938 he sustained a terrific blow on the upper part of the abdomen when he was thrown against the front seat in an automobile accident. He immediately noticed considerable pain in the upper abdominal region which he treated by abstaining from food and drinking large quantities of whiskey for the next three or four days. Although the pain became more severe, he drove from St. Louis to New Orleans for another engagement on the third day. He continued to drink whiskey even though by the fourth day he was practically doubled up with pain. On the fifth day he was operated on for a perforated ulcer, which was found on the anterior surface of the duodenum. The perforation was sutured and despite a long and stormy convalescence the patient eventually recovered.

This patient is a member of Alcoholics Anonymous (a chronic recurrent member) and has had many personal tragedies in the past eight years. He smokes to excess, when he drinks, he drinks to excess, and there are numerous periods when he pays no attention to his diet. In spite of this he has had no true ulcer recurrences.

Comment: This case illustrates the significance of trauma (both external and internal) in producing an ulcer. The blow on the abdomen was sufficient to produce a contusion of any intra-abdominal viscera. In addition to this the patient was subjected for the next four days to internal trauma in the form of large quantities of whiskey. Perforation probably occurred on the fourth day.

Case 17: E.J., a 62-year-old engineer, was first seen in 1946 with a history of exceedingly severe epigastric pain followed by vomiting of five years' duration. These attacks were unrelated to the digestive cycle and occurred at any time of the day. The pain began suddenly with no obvious cause, reached its maximum intensity rapidly and might or might not be relieved by the vomiting which usually followed shortly thereafter. Competent examinations on numerous occasions elsewhere and roentgenograms of the gastrointestinal tract consistently revealed no abnormalities. Roentgenograms of the stomach made on two occasions at the Ochsner Clinic revealed first an entirely normal stomach and, later, herniation of the pyloric mucous membrane through the pylorus into the duodenal cap. Despite a strict ulcer regimen and the use of an antispasmodic for the next month, the patient continued to have attacks with approximately the same frequency and intensity. About six weeks after we saw him he was seized with an excruciating pain in the epigastrium which continued unabated for some hours and was followed a day later by hematemesis and melena. He returned to the

Clinic, subtotal gastrectomy was performed and in addition to the herniated gastric mucosa an acute gastric ulcer was noted on the lesser curvature of the pyloric antrum near the angulus. Since the operation he has had no further gastric symptoms or hemorrhage.

Comment: This is probably a traumatic ulcer, intrinsic in origin. The acute gastric ulcer was secondary to terrific gastrospasm which in turn was caused by intussusception of gastric mucosa into the duodenum.

Case 18: P.L., a 25-year-old farmer, did not exhibit the typical ulcer characteristics although he was rather conscientious and anxious to improve himself. His ulcer symptoms began at the age of 13 years and four years later he had his first hemorrhage. There was no evidence of acute emotional disturbance or unusual traumatic or dietary factors in his history, but he did have a strong genetic background. His maternal grandfather died of "chronic stomach trouble." Two maternal uncles, one maternal aunt and one brother have proved peptic ulcers.

Comment: Although ambitious and hard working this patient did not have enough of the characteristic ulcer traits to be classified in Group A. A few questions brought out the strong genetic background and the patient himself had all the physical characteristics of Draper's constitutional ulcer type. The early onset of symptoms is typical.

Summary

For nearly a decade peptic ulcer has been widely accepted as a psychosomatic disorder. The disease is now usually considered as the end result of the interaction of constitutional, psychic, traumatic and local factors. The relationship of these factors to the personalities of a large group of patients with this disease is the basis of this monograph. Emphasis has been placed on the clinical application of recent advances in our knowledge of this psychosomatic affection. An algebraic equation is offered which we believe will aid in the understanding of the interrelation of the multiple etiologic agents involved in producing an ulcer as well as of the recurrent nature of the disorder. A series of recent cases of peptic ulcer illustrating the four groups of clinical significance is presented.

References

1. Aaron, A. H.: Personal communication.
2. Alexander, F.: The influence of psychologic factors upon gastro-intestinal disturbances; A symposium; In general principles, objectives, and preliminary results. *Psychoanalyt. Quart.* 3:501–539, Oct., 1934.
3. Alexander, F.: Personal communication.
4. Alexander, F.: Quoted by Portis, S. A.: *Diseases of the Digestive System.* Philadelphia, Lea & Febiger, 1941.
5. Alvarez, W. C.: Editorial, *Gastroenterology* 8:678, May, 1947.
6. Sullivan, A. J.: Diseases of the Stomach, p. 771 in: Blumer, G. and Sullivan, A. J.: *The Practitioner's Library of Medicine and Surgery.* Vol. VIII: Therapeutics. New York, Appleton-Century Co., 1935.
7. Blumer, G. and Sullivan, A. J.: *The Therapeutics of Internal Diseases,* Vol. III. New York, Appleton-Century Co., 1941.
8. Bonne, C. and others: Morphology of stomach and gastric secretion in Malays and Chinese and different incidence of gastric ulcer and cancer in these races. *Am. J. Cancer* 33:265–279, June, 1938.
9. Brinton, W.: *On the Pathology, Symptoms and Treatment of Ulcer of the Stomach.* John Churchill, New Burlington St., London, 1857.
10. Brown, T. R.: Treatment of peptic ulcer. *Internat. Clin.* 1:27–42, March, 1930.
11. Brown, W. T., Preu, P. W. and Sullivan, A. J.: Ulcerative colitis and the personality. *Am. J. Psychiat.* 95:407–420, Sept., 1938.
12. Brown, W.: Personal communication.
13. Crohn, B. B. and Shwartzman, G.: Ulcer recurrences attributed to upper respiratory tract infection: possible illustration of Shwartzman phenomenon. *Am. J. Digest. Dis. & Nutrition* 4:705–707, Jan., 1938.
14. Cushing, H.: Peptic ulcers and the interbrain (Balfour lecture). *Surg., Gynec. & Obst.* 55:1–34, July, 1932.
15. Davies, D. T. and Wilson, A. T. M.: Observations on life-history of chronic peptic ulcer, *Lancet* 2:1353–1360, Dec. 11, 1937.
16. Dodge, R. and Kahn, E.: *The Craving for Superiority.* New Haven, Yale Univ. Press, 1931.

93

17. Draper, G.: Emotional component of ulcer susceptible constitution. *Ann. Int. Med.* 16:633–658, April, 1942.

18. Draper, G. and Touraine, G. A.: Man-environment unit and peptic ulcer. *Arch. Int. Med.* 49:616–662, April, 1932.

19. Dunbar, H. F.: The Relationship Between Anxiety States and Organic Disease, *Clinics* 1:879–908, Dec., 1942.

20. Dunbar, H. F.: *Psychosomatic Diagnosis.* New York, Paul B. Hoeber, 1943.

21. Emery, E. S., Jr. and Monroe, R. T.: Peptic ulcer; nature and treatment based on study of 1,435 cases. *Arch. Int. Med.* 55:271–292, Feb., 1935.

22. Gainsborough, H. and Slater, E.: A study of peptic ulcer. *Brit. M. J.* 2:253–258, Aug. 24, 1946.

23. Greengard, H., Atkinson, A. J., Grossman, M. I. and Ivy, A. C.: The effectiveness of parenterally administered enterogastrone in the prophylaxis of recurrences of experimental and clinical peptic ulcer; with a summary of 58 cases. *Gastroenterology* 7:625–649, Dec., 1946.

24. Hall, G. E., Ettinger, G. H. and Banting, F. G.: Experimental production of coronary thrombosis and myocardial failure. *Canad. M. A. J.* 34:9–15, Jan., 1936.

25. Halliday, J. L.: Concept of a psychosomatic affection. *Lancet* 2:692–696, Dec. 4, 1943.

26. Halstead, J. A.: The management of "soldier's stomach" among combat infantrymen: evaluation of psychiatric and physical factors. *J. Nerv. & Ment. Dis.* 105:116–123, Feb., 1947.

26a. Friedman, M. H.: Peptic ulcer and functional dyspepsia in the armed forces. *Gastroenterology* 10:586–606, April, 1948.

27. Hurst, A. F. and Stewart, M. J.: *Gastric and Duodenal Ulcer.* With the Co-Operation in the Radiological Sections of P. J. Briggs. New York, Oxford University Press, 1929.

28. Iams, A. M. and Horton, B. T.: Ulcer which appeared in stomach of man receiving histamine intravenously. *Gastroenterology* 6:449–451, May, 1946.

29. Johnson, W.: *People in Quandaries,* New York, Harper and Brothers, 1946.

30. Jones, C. M.: Therapy of peptic ulcer from point of view of internist. *Psychosom. Med.* 8:200–204, May–June, 1946.

31. Kapp, F. T., Rosenbaum, M. and Romano, J.: Psychological factors in men with peptic ulcers. *Am. J. Psychiat.* 103:700–704, March, 1947.

32. Kaufmann, J.: Treatment of peptic ulcer. *Med. Rec.* 94:324, Aug. 24, 1918; also Tr. Am. Gastro-enterological Assoc., St. Louis, p. 19, 1918.

33. Melton, G.: Haematemesis and the war. *Lancet* 1:316–317, Feb. 17, 1940.

34. Mittelmann, B. and Wolff, H. G.: Emotions and gastroduodenal function; experimental studies on patients with gastritis, duodenitis and peptic ulcer. *Psychosom. Med.* 4:5–61, Jan., 1942.

35. Moore, F. D., Chapman, W. P., Shulz, M. D. and Jones, C. M.: Resection of the vagus nerves in peptic ulcer; physiologic effects and clinical results, with a report of two years' experience. *J. A. M. A.* 133:741–748, March 15, 1947.

36. Necheles, H.: Peptic ulcer in the Chinese. *Am. J. Digest. Dis.* 6:50–51, March, 1939.

37. Palmer, W. L.: *Portis's Diseases of the Digestive System.* Ed. 1, Philadelphia, Lea & Febiger, p. 489, 1941.

38. Price, P. B. and Lee, T. F.: The gastric digestion of living tissue. *Surg., Gynec. & Obst.* 83:61–72, July, 1946.

39. Rendle-Short, J.: Perforated peptic ulcer during air raiding. (Letter to the Editor) *Lancet* 1:429, April 4, 1942.

40. Rivers, A. B.: Clinical consideration of etiology of peptic ulcer. *Arch. Int. Med.* 53:97–119, Jan., 1934.

41. Robinson, S. C.: On etiology of peptic ulcer; analysis of 70 ulcer patients. *Am. J. Digest. Dis. & Nutrition* 2:333–343, Aug., 1935.

42. Robinson, S. C.: Role of emotions in gastroduodenal ulcers. *Illinois M. J.* 71:338–347, April, 1937.

43. Roth, J. A. and Ivy, A. C.: Caffeine and peptic ulcer. *Gastroenterology* 7:576–582, Nov., 1946.

44. Sandweiss, D. J., Saltzstein, H. C. and Farbman, A. A.: Relation of sex hormones to peptic ulcer. *Am. J. Digest. Dis. & Nutrition* 6:6–12, March, 1939.

45. Steigmann, F.: Peptic ulcer syndrome in Negro; clinical and statistical evidence on psychogenic as against racial factors in etiology of this syndrome. *Am. J. Digest. Dis. & Nutrition* 3:310–315, July, 1936.

46. Stewart, D. N. and Winser, D. M. de R.: Incidence of perforated peptic ulcer; effect of heavy air raids. *Lancet* 1:259–261, Feb. 28, 1942.

47. Sullivan, A. J. and McKell, T. E.: Personality disorders in gastroenterology. *Gastroenterology* 9:524–538, Nov., 1947.

48. Szasz, T. S., Levin, E., Kirsner, J. B. and Palmer, W. L.: The role of hostility in the pathogenesis of peptic ulcer. *Psychosom. Med.* 9:331–336, Sept.–Oct., 1947.

49. Wangensteen, O. H.: Ulcer problem; etiology with special reference to interrelationship between vascular and acid-peptic digestive factors; characterization of satisfactory operation which will protect against recurrent ulcer (Listerian oration). *Canad. M. A. J.* 53:309–331, Oct., 1945.

50. Wolf, S. and Wolff, H. G.: Evidence on genesis of peptic ulcer in man. *J. A. M. A.* 120:670–675, Oct. 31, 1942.

51. Wolf, S. and Wolff, H. G.: *Human Gastric Function.* New York, Oxford University Press, 1943.

52. Wolf, S. and Wolff, H. G.: An experimental study of changes in gastric function in response to varying life experiences. *Rev. Gastroenterol. 14*:419–434, June, 1947.

53. Zane, M. D.: Psychosomatic considerations in peptic ulcer. *Psychosom. Med. 9*:372–380, Nov.–Dec., 1947.

Index

This book

PERSONALITY
IN PEPTIC ULCER

By

ALBERT J. SULLIVAN, M.D.

THOMAS E. McKELL, M.D.

was set, printed and bound by Country Life Press Corporation of Garden City, New York. The type page is 23 x 40 picas. The page size is 5½ x 8½ inches. The cover is DuPont Fabrikoid 700–4075 Grain M-3 Pliability Medium, SB. The paper is 70 lb Ashokan coated.

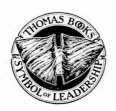

With THOMAS BOOKS *careful attention is given to all details of manufacturing and design. It is the Publisher's desire to present books that are satisfactory as to their physical qualities and artistic possibilities and appropriate for their particular use.* THOMAS BOOKS *will be true to those laws of quality that assure a good name and good will.*